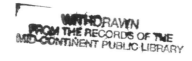

D1369529

60 Seconds to Slim

Balance Your Body Chemistry to Burn Fat Fast!

Michelle Schoffro Cook, PhD, ROHP

RODALE.

To the love of my life, Curtis

Direct hardcover first published by Rodale Inc. in January 2013.

© 2013 by Michelle Schoffro Cook

Printed in the United States of America
Rodale Inc. makes every effort to use acid-acid-free ∞, recycled paper ♻.

Book design by Chris Rhoads

Library of Congress Cataloging-in-Publication Data is on file with the publisher.

ISBN 978–1–60961–849–0   trade hardcover

2   4   6   8   10   9   7   5   3   hardcover

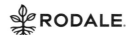

We inspire and enable people to improve their lives and the world around them.
rodalebooks.com

Contents

Acknowledgments

Curtis, thank you for all your love, support, and encouragement throughout the writing of this book and always.

Claire, thank you for your ongoing belief in my work and efforts to find a publisher for this book.

Anne, thanks for recognizing the value in this book and bringing it to the public.

Marielle, thanks for your vision and efforts to make *60 Seconds to Slim* the book it is. And thanks for being such a pleasure to work with.

Thanks to everyone else at Rodale for all your efforts to edit, package, promote, and market my book.

Thanks to the many people who shared their stories, measurements, weight, and personal details to help people know how well this program works.

Thanks to the people who provided recipes, namely Cobi Slater, PhD, DNM, CHT, RNCP, ROHP; Angela Grow; and Denise Passerello, MS, CPT, CNC.

Thanks to my parents, Michael and Deborah Schoffro, for your love and support throughout the years.

Introduction

A Pandemic Problem

In the modern world, humans are unhealthier than ever and our harmful choices and environment are causing us to tip the scales as never before. By 2015, 75 percent of the American population will be overweight and 41 percent will be obese (meaning they will be more than 20 percent heavier than the ideal weight for their height), according to Reuters.[1] That means 187.5 million Americans will be overweight or obese just 2 years from now. And there's more: In the last year alone, obesity rates rose in 16 American states.[2] The remaining states continued to have the same high obesity rates. Not one state had a decline. Scary.

The situation in Canada isn't much different: 23 percent of adults are obese. And Europeans and Asians are experiencing a growing obesity problem as well, with the percentage of overweight or obese children there tripling in the last three decades.

According to a study by the United States Centers for Disease Control and Prevention (CDC), being overweight is directly linked to at least 20 health conditions, including heart disease and diabetes.[3] The overweight and obesity problem is serious. Adult diabetes rates increased in 11 states and Washington, DC, in the past year. In eight states, more than 10 percent of adults have type 2 diabetes.[4] Some of the complications linked to diabetes include blindness, limb amputation, severe infection, coma, and death.

Considering the exponential rise in weight issues, it may come as no surprise that, in my more than two decades of experience as a nutritionist and natural health consultant, increasing numbers of clients have asked me the best way to lose weight. In that time, I've seen many fad diets come and go. While some included high amounts of fat, others eliminated fat altogether. Some diets recommended large amounts of protein while others suggested only vegetarian foods. Some diets deprived people of carbohydrates while others allowed certain types of carbs.

Today's fad diets focus primarily on low-carb, no-carb, and high-protein regimens. But, regardless of the diet craze, they share a few traits.

1. They typically work well in the short term, until the dieters relax their strict guidelines and gain back the weight—sometimes even more than they started out with.
2. They do not include enough food to sustain a person for any length of time. And they don't include a wide enough variety of food and enough calories to provide adequate nutrition to maintain health.
3. They claim that the diet works for everyone, no matter a person's metabolism, genetic predispositions, eating habits, or lifestyle. These one-size-fits-all diets mislead consumers with unrealistic promises.
4. They can cause potentially damaging long-term consequences, like fatigue, irritability, and even possible organ damage, particularly to the kidneys and liver.
5. They do not consider people from a holistic perspective: body, mind, emotions, and spirit. All these different facets can play a role in whether a person becomes or stays heavy.

I knew there had to be a better way to lose weight: an approach that worked in the short term but could be continued for life; one that ensured an adequate variety and quantity of nutrients to help keep people healthy for life; a diet that recognized inherent variations in habits and lifestyles so it allowed flexibility; and one that would not damage the body but would ensure greater health, vitality, immunity, and wellness while addressing people from a holistic viewpoint.

60 Seconds to Slim is the culmination of 2 decades of research and clinical experience learning what works, what doesn't, and what only appears to work for a little while. It seeks to balance your inner terrain: your biochemistry, energy, emotions, and more—but we'll get to that momentarily.

My 20-year search for the secret to healthy weight loss confirmed that balancing pH is critical. Additionally, strengthening the body's liver, lymphatic system, intestinal flora balance, emotional well-being, and thyroid and adrenal health are all components of the program I'll be sharing with you in this book. Even if you're not familiar with any of these terms, they will soon become second nature.

Serving Up a Plan with My Vision and Values

After detailing the natural and effective weight-loss approach I fine-tuned over time, I am happy to report that I had an almost immediate response from publishers interested in *60 Seconds to Slim*. Some wanted to turn it into the dieting equivalent of the get-rich-quick scheme. You know, the ones that promise you'll lose weight at a furious pace but neglect to tell you that you'll gain it all back and more if you don't remain ever vigilant in eating next to nothing. They're the ones that promise you'll be skinnier than a rake and forget to tell you that it is nearly impossible to get all the nutrients you need to maintain strong bones and a healthy immune system on their plan. They also neglect to tell you that you may turn into a cranky, miserable version of yourself when your hormones become imbalanced because of insufficient hormone building blocks. To sign one of these book deals would have required me to sacrifice not only the vision I had for this book but my personal ethics as well—something I was not prepared to do in exchange for a book contract.

One publisher immediately loved the book but insisted the title must be changed to *60 Seconds to Skinny*. I felt my heart sink. I couldn't do it. To some people, it was only a single word change, but to me it was so much more. To me, the word *skinny* implies thinness taken to the extreme. While some people are naturally skinny, many people—especially women—strive for a weight that is neither attainable nor healthy for their frame. Many other weight-loss books capitalize on people's desire to become skinny at any cost, including their health, but that's not an approach I am comfortable with.

I knew only too well how women (and men) fall prey to these types of diets. When I was 14, I suffered from anorexia and dropped below 60 pounds. Like many young women, I nearly lost my life striving to reach model-thin proportions and airbrushed, cover girl perfection. The fashion and weight-loss industries promote "models" who, ironically, are anything but healthy models for women. These industries glorify more of a caricature than an attractive ideal. Yet many women, myself included, have fallen prey to their message that "there is no such thing as too skinny." Actually, there is. The epidemic of eating disorders and the many people who lose their lives or their sense of self in an effort to become skinny prove that there *is* such a thing as too skinny.

So, if you're looking for a book to help you lose as much weight as possible as fast as possible at any cost, *60 Seconds to Slim* is not the book for you. But if you are looking to lose weight because you would like to be at a healthy weight for your frame and body type while feeling better than ever (just by making a few simple, 60-second changes to your regular routine), then you have come to the right place. If you are looking for a healthy way to lose excessive pounds and to achieve a weight that feels right for you and is not based on an arbitrary number, keep reading. If you're looking for a program that recognizes the physical, as well as the emotional, aspects of weight, then *60 Seconds to Slim* is your program.

A Tested Program Designed with YOU in Mind

60 Seconds to Slim is based on the program I developed for my clients and use in my health practice. When a client first comes to see me about weight issues, of course we explore the foods she is eating and isn't eating, but we also explore what was happening in her life when she first started to gain more weight than she wants to carry on her body. We examine her goals and the reasons why she wants to lose weight.

Some people may find value in the militaristic "boot camp" approach to weight management, but I am not one of them; therefore, the approach I take with clients (and now, readers) includes being kind to yourself while finding new ways to comfort yourself in stressful times that do not include emotional eating. It involves learning new ways to prepare food so you have all the enjoyment and pleasure food can offer without inflicting damage on your body. It includes learning to love yourself and your body, rather than allowing it to be treated like dirt—the way many weight-loss boot camp gurus treat their clients. It also involves taking responsibility for your choices.

60 Seconds to Slim is based on a natural approach to healing that I call pHytozyme therapy. That's because I work with people to balance their body chemistry (pH), increase the phytonutrient-rich food in their diet, and improve their enzyme systems. Don't worry if you're not familiar with these concepts or terms. I'll be explaining them throughout this book, and we'll work together to improve all these elements that lead to natural, healthy weight loss throughout the 60 Seconds to Slim Plan.

One of the main differences between my approach to weight loss and many other programs is time. As a busy health professional, author, blogger, and e-publisher, I find that time is the resource most at a premium in my life. And I know I am no different from most other people out there. Statistics show that people are busier than ever: working more hours than previous generations to make ends meet, with more demands on their time.

Formerly, my clients would complain that they didn't have time to eat well or exercise. While I don't necessarily agree that it takes any longer to eat healthier than to eat poorly if you learn some simple tricks, most people don't know them. The same is true for exercise: It is easy to adopt a lifestyle that includes exercise without necessarily finding an hour to lock yourself up in a health club—not that there is anything wrong with that if you enjoy it. But exercise simply isn't enjoyable to most people unless they learn how to have fun with it.

The main point of *60 Seconds to Slim* is that you don't need to devote your whole life to attaining a healthy weight. Weight loss is more likely to happen if you stop stressing over it and make simple (but better) choices for your diet and lifestyle. Most of these changes take less than a minute to implement but have profound health and weight-loss effects. And better yet, I've included only tips and techniques that are seriously beneficial. That way, you won't waste time on methods that don't work. Instead, you'll lose weight, your energy and confidence will soar, you'll reduce the harmful effects of aging, you'll prevent disease, and you'll feel better than ever.

I know that sounds like a tall order, but when you work within the body's requirements for health, weight melts off without the effort. Your body isn't conspiring to make you fat. Conversely, your body wants you to feed it the foods and nutrients it needs to create the healthiest you possible, and at the healthiest weight. The same is true when you make healthy lifestyle choices: Your body has the elements it needs to make healthier cells, tissues, organs, and organ systems. And that spells a healthier weight and a healthier you.

How to Use This Book

60 Seconds to Slim is divided into three parts. In Part I, you'll discover the importance of balancing your body chemistry, or more specifically, your pH levels. (You don't need to be familiar with pH. I'll explain everything you need to understand how to balance your weight by eliminating acid from your body.) Then I'll share with you the essential 60 Seconds to Slim Plan that forms the foundation of this program. You'll continue to follow the basic tenets laid out in Chapter 2 as long as you are trying to lose weight.

In Part II, you'll be introduced to the simple 60-Second Weight-Loss Tips that will help you maximize your weight-loss efforts. Rest assured that you don't need to follow them *all* to get results—although you can if you want to, and doing so will only serve you better.

Finally, in Part III, I give you delicious recipes designed specifically to help you achieve success on this program. They are easy and fun to make, feature all kinds of cuisine, and most important, deliver beneficial nutrients and restore your body's pH.

Contrary to what you may believe, addressing excess weight or obesity doesn't have to be a battle. By making healthier choices that include eating foods rich in phytonutrients, balancing your body chemistry, stabilizing your blood sugar, reinforcing your diet with a few carefully selected supplements, and doing the right kind of exercise, you can maintain your weight loss over the long term. Don't worry if that sounds hard—it's not. I'm going to guide you step-by-step in making the best choices to lose weight and keep it off. And those choices will take 60 seconds or less.

60 SECONDS TO SLIM
AT A GLANCE

THE ESSENTIAL PLAN: Follow these basic guidelines for eating a more alkaline diet and incorporating exercise to jump-start your weight loss and prime your body for success when adding the 60-Second Tips.

Week 1: **SUBSTITUTE** In Chapter 3, you'll learn about the foods and ingredients that are sabotaging your efforts to be slim and healthy and how to replace them with better options. Be sure to make *all* of the recommended substitutions in this week, because, as you'll learn, eliminating those ingredients and toxins is essential if you want to see results.

Week 2: **BOOST** In Chapter 4, you'll learn about the most important fat-burning foods and how to add them to your diet. Choose at least five of the recommended weight-loss boosters this week to add to your routine.

Week 3: **STRATEGIZE** In Chapter 5, you'll learn about the scientifically proven timing tricks and fat-burning strategies that will supercharge your body's pH-balancing abilities, balance its hormonal mechanisms, power up your metabolism, and improve the detoxification pathways that burn fat. Choose at least five of the recommended weight-loss strategies this week.

Week 4: **SUPPLEMENT** In Chapter 6, you'll learn about the proven weight-loss nutrients and remedies that will support your body's metabolism and help you burn fat, while improving your health. You'll also learn ways to determine which supplements are right for you and which you can skip. Choose at least two of the recommended weight-loss supplements this week, in addition to any supplements you may already be taking.

PART 1

THE ACID-ALKALINE
CONNECTION

Chapter 1

Managing Your Acid Levels

You may not realize it, but you—and most other humans today—are coping with a problem not unlike the acid rain problem trees face. You are probably familiar with acid rain and its ravages. Laden with toxic pollutants and emissions, acid rain has a damaging effect on trees, harming their ability to withstand pests, disease, drought, and cold. It can even prevent a plant from reproducing. To combat acidity and stay alive, the tree or plant must pull minerals such as calcium and magnesium from the soil. But over time, the soil becomes depleted of these minerals, reducing the tree's chances of survival.

Modern humans are very much like those trees. When we eat a highly acid-forming diet, it is comparable to creating acid rain in our bloodstreams. In the same way we've polluted our planet, we are unconsciously polluting our bodies, which are basically microcosms of the natural world. The main difference is that we are well aware that we are polluting Mother Earth, but few people recognize that our bodies are suffering from internal pollution and acid waste. Fewer still recognize that internal pollution and acidity are linked to weight gain and obesity.

Our bodies must maintain an internal balance between acidity on one side of the spectrum and alkalinity on the other. This spectrum is known as the pH scale. Imagine that the pH scale is like a tug-of-war in your body. On one side is the acid team and on the other side is the alkaline team. The middle is neutral, which reads 7.0 on the scale between 0 (extremely acidic) and 14.0 (extremely alkaline). Most of what we eat and our lifestyle choices tip the balance in favor of acidity and also contribute to weight gain. Yet our blood needs to remain stable at 7.365 (slightly alkaline) to maintain health and life.

We cannot live if our body becomes acidic, so the body has mechanisms in place to ensure that the blood, which feeds our brain and all our organs, glands, and tissues, remains slightly alkaline. The body, in its infinite wisdom, has many ways to deal with acidity, but one of the ways we're concerned with is the tendency to store acid in fat cells to get it out of the blood quickly. Fat cells are your body's natural buffer against acid since they have a natural affinity for acidic toxins and acidic by-products of metabolism. Fat is actually your body's ally against acidic food choices, although I know more than a few people will find it hard to believe that fat is helpful to the body.

As an example, let's look at one of the most acid-forming foods we eat: sugar. When you eat sugar, it ferments in your body, forming lactic acid that, if not eliminated, will break down cells and lead to disease. In an effort to combat the acidity, your body goes into preservation mode and uses the fat in your diet and in your body to buffer and neutralize the acid. It attempts to eliminate the fat from your body, but if this is not possible, it will store it as fat deposits to keep the acid out of the bloodstream and away from organs, where it can do damage. If the acid is not eliminated, it will damage cells and tissues, leading to a breakdown of tissues, bones, and organs in the body.[1]

Acidity can also impair the proper functioning of our hormonal systems, which I probably don't have to tell you can cause weight gain. You'll learn more about this in some of the 60-Second Weight-Loss Tips later in this book.

Meat, dairy products, sugary foods, soda, coffee, and many other foods are all extremely acidifying to the body. Yet they are exactly what most people eat on a daily basis. Reducing the amount of acidic food in favor of alkaline choices gives your body a chance to restore balance at the cellular level, which allows it to start breaking down fat stores and ultimately rebalance your weight. But before we get to that, let's first take a closer look at acidity and alkalinity, why you need to prevent your body from becoming excessively acidic, and the weight-loss benefits of balancing your body chemistry.

Kick the Acid Out

If you've poured vinegar and baking soda in your sink to unclog the drain, you are already familiar with the pH concept, even if you didn't realize it. Vinegar is acidic and baking soda is alkaline. When mixed together, they bubble and fizz to neutralize each other. This is the whole foundation of the pH scale.

The term *pH* stands for "potential of hydrogen," which means the amount of hydrogen in a solution. But it isn't necessary to understand hydrogen atoms or hold a degree in biochemistry to grasp this concept. As I mentioned above, the scale ranges from 0, which is extremely acidic, to 14.0, which is extremely alkaline, with neutral being 7.0, in the middle of the spectrum.

Most of our bodily tissues need to be slightly alkaline for optimum health and weight. Your blood also needs to be slightly alkaline to keep you alive. Blood nourishes your organs, organ systems, tissues, and cells. Our primary goal throughout *60 Seconds to Slim* will be to balance your body chemistry to ensure that your body and its cells, tissues, and organs are nourished.

Our biggest battle in overcoming acidity is our addiction to what I call the Standard American Diet (SAD). I'll get back to this topic in a moment. Our second biggest battle, and one that goes hand in hand with our SAD eating habits, is the stressful lifestyles many of us feel we cannot control. Poor food choices and stress push us toward the acidic side of the pH spectrum, causing our body to expend its resources on managing continuous—or chronic— acidity. Keep in mind that this imbalance is not the same thing as metabolic acidosis, a serious condition that can occur in relation to a preexisting disease and that requires hospitalization and medical treatment. I am talking about the ongoing, gradual, and accumulating impacts of this imbalance that manifest in numerous nagging physical and emotional symptoms, including weight gain as well as increasing vulnerability to disease.

Are You Acidic?

There are numerous ways to find out if you're acidic. In our modern world, the vast majority of people, even most health-conscious people, are acidic. I've developed a quiz to help you understand many of the factors that contribute to acidity. While it is not the same as testing your urine or saliva, it still gives you a good basis from which to work. Afterward, I'll explain how to test your urine or saliva pH to get an even better perspective on your acid-alkaline balance, or lack thereof.

So before we dive further into the 60 Seconds to Slim program, let's assess your current dietary and lifestyle habits, particularly to learn how they may be contributing to excess acidity and fat in your body. Here is the quiz I regularly use with my clients. Grab a pencil and paper to keep track of your points—and remember: Be honest!

Diet and Lifestyle

1. I add sugar or artificial sweeteners to tea, coffee, cereal, or other food or drinks

    ○ 2 or more times a day (5 points)
    ○ Once a day (4 points)
    ○ 3 to 6 times a week (3 points)
    ○ Once or twice a week (2 points)
    ○ Less than once a week (1 point)
    ○ Never (0 points)

2. I eat fried foods (including battered chicken and fish, french fries, fried packaged foods, etc.)

    ○ 2 or more times a day (5 points)
    ○ Once a day (4 points)
    ○ 3 to 6 times a week (3 points)
    ○ Once or twice a week (2 points)
    ○ Less than once a week (1 point)
    ○ Never (0 points)

3. I eat desserts (cake, cookies, doughnuts, pies, etc.) and drink sweetened drinks (including sports drinks, iced tea, lemonade, and bottled fruit juices)

    ○ 2 or more times a day (5 points)
    ○ Once a day (4 points)
    ○ 3 to 6 times a week (3 points)
    ○ Once or twice a week (2 points)
    ○ Less than once a week (1 point)
    ○ Never (0 points)

4. I drink cola or other soda (any kind, regular or diet)

    ○ 2 or more times a day (6 points)
    ○ Once a day (5 points)
    ○ 3 to 6 times a week (4 points)
    ○ Once or twice a week (3 points)
    ○ Less than once a week (2 points)
    ○ Never (0 points)

(continued on the next page)

5. **I eat fast food (burgers, fries, onion rings, tacos, pizza, submarine sandwiches, etc.)**
   - ○ 2 or more times a day (5 points)
   - ○ Once a day (4 points)
   - ○ 3 to 6 times a week (3 points)
   - ○ Once or twice a week (2 points)
   - ○ Less than once a week (1 point)
   - ○ Never (0 points)

6. **I eat convenience store snacks (chocolate bars, chips, Slurpees, etc.)**
   - ○ 2 or more times a day (5 points)
   - ○ Once a day (4 points)
   - ○ 3 to 6 times a week (3 points)
   - ○ Once or twice a week (2 points)
   - ○ Less than once a week (1 point)
   - ○ Never (0 points)

7. **I drink or eat dairy products (milk, cheese, ice cream, yogurt, etc.)**
   - ○ 2 or more times a day (4 points)
   - ○ Once a day (3 points)
   - ○ 3 to 6 times a week (2 points)
   - ○ Once or twice a week (1 point)
   - ○ Less than once a week (1 point)
   - ○ Never (0 points)

8. **I eat processed, packaged foods (boxed cereals, microwaveable meals, canned soups and sauces, TV dinners, etc.)**
   - ○ 2 or more times a day (5 points)
   - ○ Once a day (4 points)
   - ○ 3 to 6 times a week (3 points)
   - ○ Once or twice a week (2 points)
   - ○ Less than once a week (1 point)
   - ○ Never (0 points)

9. **I eat red meat and/or pork**
   - ○ 2 or more times a day (5 points)
   - ○ Once a day (4 points)
   - ○ 3 to 6 times a week (3 points)
   - ○ Once or twice a week (2 points)
   - ○ Less than once a week (1 point)
   - ○ Never (0 points)

10. **I eat chicken and/or fish (not fried or battered)**
    - ○ 2 or more times a day (3 points)
    - ○ Once a day (2 points)
    - ○ 3 to 6 times a week (1 point)
    - ○ Once or twice a week (1 point)
    - ○ Less than once a week (1 point)
    - ○ Never (0 points)

11. **I smoke cigarettes**
- ○ 2 or more times a day (5 points)
- ○ Once a day (4 points)
- ○ 3 to 6 times a week (3 points)
- ○ Once or twice a week (2 points)
- ○ Less than once a week (1 point)
- ○ Never (0 points)

12. **I drink alcohol as follows**
- ○ 2 or more glasses of wine, beer, or other alcoholic beverage a day (5 points)
- ○ 1 glass of wine, bottle of beer, or other alcoholic beverage a day (4 points)
- ○ 3 to 6 times a week (3 points)
- ○ Once or twice a week (2 points)
- ○ Less than once a week (1 point)
- ○ Never (0 points)

13. **I take over-the-counter or prescription medications**
- ○ 2 or more times a day, or more than one medication (5 points)
- ○ Once a day (4 points)
- ○ 3 to 6 times a week (3 points)
- ○ Once or twice a week (2 points)
- ○ Less than once a week (1 point)
- ○ Never (0 points)

14. **I feel stressed about my life/job/ relationship**
- ○ 2 or more times a day (5 points)
- ○ Once a day (4 points)
- ○ 3 to 6 times a week (3 points)
- ○ Once or twice a week (2 points)
- ○ Less than once a week (1 point)
- ○ Never (0 points)

15. **I use nonorganic personal care products like shampoo, deodorant, or perfume and chemical household cleaning products**
- ○ 2 or more times a day (3 points)
- ○ Once a day (2 points)
- ○ 3 to 6 times a week (2 points)
- ○ Once or twice a week (1 point)
- ○ Less than once a week (1 point)
- ○ Never (0 points)

16. **I eat pastries, breads, cereals, or baked goods containing white flour**
- ○ 2 or more times a day (5 points)
- ○ Once a day (4 points)
- ○ 3 to 6 times a week (3 points)
- ○ Once or twice a week (2 points)
- ○ Less than once a week (1 point)
- ○ Never (0 points)

Section A Total: _____

(continued on the next page)

section b

Symptoms and Disease

Give yourself 3 points for every symptom or illness below that you experience on an ongoing (daily) basis and any disease or disorder you have been diagnosed with; 2 points for every symptom or illness you experience frequently (weekly); 1 point for every symptom or illness you experience infrequently (1 to 2 times a year); and 0 points if you don't experience the symptom or illness at all.

___Allergies, asthma, other respiratory concerns

___Alzheimer's disease, Parkinson's disease, senility, dementia, other brain disorders

___Arteriosclerosis, heart disease, heart attack, stroke, high cholesterol

___Arthritis, gout, ankylosing spondylitis

___Bronchitis, tonsillitis, laryngitis, other respiratory infections

___Cancer

___Chronic fatigue syndrome (diagnosed by a doctor), fibromyalgia, environmental illness

___Colds or flu infections more than once a year (give yourself 0 points if once per year or less often)

___Depression

___Diabetes

___Difficulty gaining weight

___Digestive concerns: pain, indigestion, constipation, diarrhea, heartburn, irritable bowel syndrome, colitis

___Gynecological problems such as yeast infections, endometriosis, premenstrual syndrome, menopausal symptoms, etc.

___Headaches or migraines

___Hormonal imbalances

___Kidney disease or urinary tract infections

___Multiple sclerosis, muscular dystrophy

___Muscle loss, cramping, or wasting

___Osteoporosis, bone density loss, fractures or bone breaks

___Pain or discomfort

___Premature aging or graying

___Prostate problems

___Sinusitis or rhinitis

___Tooth decay, loss of teeth

___Weight gain, obesity, difficulty losing weight

Section B Total: _____

Section A + Section B Total: _____

Healthy Living

I suspect most people are horrified and dismayed when they tally up their score. I'm going to give you a chance to improve it without cheating. Simply calculate your score for the questions below:

1. **I eat raw vegetables**
   - ○ 4 or more times a day (4 points)
   - ○ 2 or 3 times a day (2 points)
   - ○ Once a day (1 points)
   - ○ Less than once a day (0 points)

2. **I drink filtered water or alkaline water**
   - ○ 10 cups or more a day (4 points)
   - ○ 7 to 9 cups a day (2 points)
   - ○ 4 to 7 cups a day (1 point)
   - ○ Less than 4 cups a day (0 points)

3. **I exercise for at least 30 minutes (including walking at least 10,000 steps)**
   - ○ Every day (4 points)
   - ○ 4 to 6 times a week (3 points)
   - ○ 2 to 3 times a week (2 points)
   - ○ Once a week (1 point)
   - ○ Less than once a week (0 points)

4. **I take time for myself (meditation, rest, relaxation of at least 30 minutes)**
   - ○ Every day (4 points)
   - ○ 4 to 6 times a week (3 points)
   - ○ 2 to 3 times a week (2 points)
   - ○ Once a week (1 point)
   - ○ Less than once a week (0 points)

Section C Total: _____

After you total your score for these questions, subtract this number from your Section A + B total. Did it reduce your total? Turn the page to learn what your score means.

Final Score

○ **Over 50:** Danger zone. Your body is dealing with chronic high levels of acidity and will rarely have a balanced pH unless it robs your bones, tissues, and organs of existing stores of alkaline substances. Your health may be in danger, and acidity is likely playing a major role in any excess weight you might be experiencing. The time for change is now. It's not too late to balance your body chemistry and start reaping the rewards. Read on!

○ **35 to 50:** Warning alarms are sounding. Your diet and lifestyle are too acidic. You may already be experiencing symptoms of an imbalanced pH, such as fatigue, infections, inflammation, digestive problems, excess weight, and allergies. You are probably eating the textbook Standard American Diet. If so, you need to address diet and lifestyle issues to decrease your exposure to acidic foods and habits that may be contributing to excess weight and potential health issues. *60 Seconds to Slim* will show you how.

○ **20 to 34:** You probably feel you live a fairly healthy lifestyle. Compared to most North Americans, you do. But your diet is probably still too acidic for your body's needs, and you may be paying a price for your choices, even if you haven't started to experience symptoms yet. Read on to learn how to make your "healthy lifestyle" healthier.

○ **10 to 19:** You are well on your way toward balancing your biochemistry. Sure, you have moments of weakness, but overall you are giving your body a fighting chance to maintain a slightly alkaline condition. If all your points came from one or two areas, you already know what you need to do. *60 Seconds to Slim* will help you fine-tune your lifestyle for optimum weight and health.

○ **Under 10:** This is the pH equivalent of Mensa. Very few people will find themselves in this range. If your score is this low, congratulations. However, if you are overweight, you may still benefit from additional effort to balance your pH and address other factors that may be affecting your weight. *60 Seconds to Slim* will teach you how to tip the pH scales back into balance for those times when you *are* too acidic. Additionally, we'll explore other factors that may be contributing to your weight.

Now that you have a sense of where you stand on the pH scale, it's time to start tracking your pH. This is an eye-opening exercise for most people.

What Is a Balanced pH?

You learned above that your blood needs to maintain a slightly alkaline pH reading of 7.365, but don't let the small numbers fool you. A change in pH from 7.0 to 6.0 equates to a tenfold increase in acidity. To regain a pH of 7.0, approximately 20 times as much alkaline substance is required. Because the SAD approach to food is so acid forming, you can see how hard it is to overcome acidity without adopting new eating strategies. And overcoming acidity doesn't mean becoming as alkaline as possible—that leads to a host of different health problems. Again, the eating habits and highly stressful lives most people lead prevent them from ever having an overly alkaline or base pH.

There are a variety of ways to test your pH, which I'll discuss in detail momentarily, but most people find saliva testing to be the easiest. Take a piece of pH test paper—available in most health food stores—and place it under your tongue briefly, then compare it with the color chart on the back of the package. You may be surprised how acidic your pH actually is.

Ironically, saliva testing that indicates an overly alkaline pH is also typically a sign of acidity and reflective of the body taking action to counter the high-acid pH. I know this seems counterintuitive, but bear with me while I explain. For example, Joe's SAD habits lead to a daily consumption of hamburgers, potato chips, milk, pie, and cola. These are acidic foods and they create an acidic imbalance that Joe's body immediately tries to correct by releasing alkaline substances from organs, bones, and tissues. Measuring pH when this is happening might show an alkaline condition because Joe's body has responded to excessive acidity. However, the ongoing need to counter this acidic onslaught takes a toll on Joe's body. He may not be experiencing negative symptoms of his SAD choices yet; however, his pH is not balanced, and it is only a matter of time before health concerns such as weight gain or fatigue affect him.

Remember, when your body is forced to deal with a highly acidic diet, your blood has to do the heavy lifting. I will refer to this condition as "acidic blood," even though, from a medical perspective, your blood cannot actually become acidic based on dietary choices. You would die long before acidic blood ran through your veins. Your body, in its infinite wisdom, does everything it can to regulate acidity and keep your blood in that slim alkaline range. As if being on the job 24/7 weren't enough, the body's efforts are often complicated by our food and drink choices. Even shallow breathing, lack of exercise, or exposure to unhealthy substances (pollution, chemicals, and fake fragrances we put on our skin or in our hair, for example) can throw off our pH balance and increase our acidity. Our body tries to store excess acid in our tissues, which decreases their pH. Our blood attempts to compensate by pulling minerals stored in our body to increase our alkalinity. Continual imbalances in the blood's pH make it less effective at neutralizing and eliminating acidity and waste products from the body. As these toxins persist and accumulate in the body, the potential for disease increases, as does the likelihood of weight gain or obesity.

How to Test Your Body's pH

Testing your pH is not critical. But I highly recommend it since it tends to be an eye-opener for most people, particularly if done regularly. In all likelihood, as is true of the vast majority of the population, your body is acidic and the most important thing you can do is to start implementing the changes you find in this book and eating the delicious recipes. Still, inquiring minds want to know, so I will explain a few methods available to get a reasonable idea of where you stand. You can check your body's acidity with saliva, urine, or blood tests. Despite the claims of some manufacturers, saliva tests are not as effective as urine tests; however, you may not be interested in dealing with urine, and who can blame you? The saliva test will give a good approximation of how acid or alkaline you are and allow you to easily check your pH over time. This is beneficial to help you identify trends or changes as you improve your diet and lifestyle.

Saliva Testing

As I mentioned above, saliva testing provides you with a rough guide to the pH of your saliva, which in turn gives you general information about your overall acid-alkaline balance. It is the easiest and least expensive way to monitor your pH. Check your local health food store for pH paper, which comes in a small roll and usually costs less than $15. A roll will last a long time when you use an inch or two for each test, allowing you to check your saliva hundreds of times.

If you have ever checked a pool or hot tub for water quality, you will understand the basic concept of pH paper. It changes color when it gets wet, and you compare it with the color-coded chart on the package. To test your saliva, hold one end of the strip and place the other end under your tongue in some saliva. The test works best if the paper does not touch your lips or tongue on the way in. A couple of seconds in your mouth are enough. After removing the paper, check its color against the chart immediately. You will probably find the reading lands between 6.0 and 8.0. Remember, the lower number is acidic, the higher number is alkaline, and our goal is slightly alkaline, or about 7.3.

Testing your saliva works best when you have not had anything to eat or drink within an hour of testing. Testing after you've eaten will affect the accuracy of the readings since your body will secrete alkaline substances in your saliva that will give you a false impression of alkalinity, even if your body is actually acidic. That's why it's best to test first thing in the morning or at least an hour after eating. Testing yourself every morning when you first wake up will help you keep an accurate account of your body's pH level and identify trends. Daily testing is important at first because if you regularly test yourself and obtain acidic readings with only rare alkaline readings, it means your body may be dumping alkaline minerals from your muscles and bones to compensate for a very acidic body and the very acidic diet it is being fed. After a week or two, you may just want to test yourself weekly.

Urine Testing

If you wish to try urine testing, you will also be relying on pH paper, placing it in the urine stream as you go to the bathroom. Alternatively, you can collect some urine in a cup and dip the pH paper strip into it. The same rule applies to urine testing—it's best conducted first thing in the morning. Urine usually tests slightly more acidic than saliva, and while urine testing is more accurate than saliva testing, the results should still be considered a guideline rather than gospel.

Blood Testing

While blood testing is the most accurate way of measuring your pH, it still provides only a snapshot of your blood's acid-alkaline balance at a specific time on one day. These tests are performed by medical personnel and sent to laboratories for analysis, so they are more costly and less convenient than the tests mentioned above. Additionally, blood tests may show up as alkaline, but your body may have taken extreme measures, like buffering acid in fat stores or pulling minerals out of muscles or bones, so that the blood will appear normal.

What Do the Results Mean?

The first thing you need to keep in mind when checking the results of your pH test is that an abundance of misinformation is available to the public. Whether you look for answers on the Internet, in books, or at your local health food store, you will inevitably encounter contradictory information and instructions. Even the companies that manufacture the pH products can disagree with each other. I have done my best to analyze the research for you and to eliminate the doubt and differing opinions. You need to know this: Your saliva pH should be between 7.0 and 7.4. Your urine pH should be around 6.8.

As you test yourself over time, you may find that your results vary—sometimes you test quite alkaline, while at other times, you seem very acidic. Earlier in this chapter, I mentioned that your body naturally does what it can to restore acid-alkaline balance. An acidic test (6.3, for example) on a regular basis with an occasional high-alkaline test may be evidence of your body dumping minerals from bones and tissues to overcome acidity. I would conclude that you are generally acidic in this scenario even though you have some alkaline readings. Similarly, if you always seem to have a high-alkaline test (let's say 8.0), I would conclude that your body is continually dumping minerals to offset excess acidity.

I've had many clients brag how alkaline their bodies are, telling me that they regularly test around 8.0 or just under. That's not a healthy state to be in either. Your body continually strives for balance and, to get your blood to a healthy 7.365 pH, it will sometimes take drastic measures. If your body's pH level rises too high, it is usually evidence that something is wrong. Excessive alkalinity can be just as harmful as excess acidity. When someone is regularly testing around 8.0, that is usually a sign that she is extremely acidic and her body is dumping alkaline minerals and nutrients from her bones or muscles to counterbalance the acidity.

Testing your pH provides you with a snapshot of your acid-alkaline balance at the moment you conduct the test. I have found that many of my clients are motivated by the test strip. They see it as visible, tangible evidence of an important aspect of their health. Alternatively, you may be the type of person who can measure results by how you feel. After you have eaten an alkaline diet for a few days, tune in to your energy level: Has it increased? When was the last time you felt bloated or experienced heartburn? Has your sleep improved? What about pain levels, allergy symptoms, nagging injuries, or infections? Have you seen positive results in these areas? They may be easier to notice over time.

Although I encourage you to test your pH before starting this program, testing is not essential. Even if you are the healthiest person you know, your diet is likely acidic and you will benefit immensely from a few simple, delicious changes to your eating habits. Later in *60 Seconds to Slim,* I will introduce you to fantastic foods and recipes for a low-acid, high-alkaline diet that supports healthy weight loss and increased vitality. And while you won't be able to see what's going on inside you, you will have taken a load off your body's internal acid-fighting mechanisms, reducing your exposure to stress and disease.

Stress and Acidity

We all experience way too much stress. In fact, most people leading modern lives are dealing with high levels of chronic stress. It has become a way of life and, disturbingly, a badge of honor for some people who boast about being overworked and close to the breaking point. On top of all this unnatural stress, many people have become adrenaline junkies, which, as the name implies, is an addiction to the rush they get from extreme sports or other stress-filled activities.

Stress, including the self-inflicted adrenaline rushes that have become synonymous with "fun," will cause damage to the body. Stress causes both an increased level of acidity and weight gain. When your body is stressed in any way, it pumps out hormones to manage the situation. We are still animals, and our bodies cannot differentiate the stress we have on the job from the stress of running away from a grizzly bear. The hormonal release sends more blood to your limbs—even at the expense of your brain—and accelerates your breathing in preparation for a battle or a rapid escape. This is the primal fight-or-flight response that humans share with other animals. We need it to ensure escape from danger but it doesn't necessarily help us deal with being cut off in traffic, being yelled at by our boss, or coping with spoiled, screaming children.

We need these hormones to do their job, but they were never intended to be secreted continuously to deal with the pressures of modern living. In these situations of chronic stress, the hormones will make your body more acidic. Additionally, we tend to take rapid, shallow breaths when we are stressed, causing our oxygen uptake to decrease. Oxygen alkalizes the blood, which nourishes the body's tissues and organs. Less oxygen leads to more acidity. Breathing is one of our body's ways of trying to maintain an alkaline balance, but we need to breathe deeply and inhale oxygen-rich air to benefit from it.

Toxins and Acidity

Humans have always had to deal with toxic substances in their environment— they form naturally in the air, water, and soil, and our bodies have mechanisms in place to manage many of these exposures. Unfortunately, the human body was not designed to deal with the tens of thousands of chemicals used on a daily basis on this planet, including thousands of toxic substances that contaminate our food, air, and water.

Over a decade ago, in 2000, an estimated 4 billion pounds of chemicals were released into the ground and another 2 billion pounds of chemical emissions were pumped into the atmosphere. These numbers are not decreasing as the years go by. Even more disturbing is the fact that these are only the toxins being monitored or tracked. Countless others have neither been identified nor are being measured. In Canada, the National Research Council reports that it has no toxicity data on more than 80 percent of the chemicals in commercial use because their impact on the human body has not been studied. These are toxins that end up in the water we drink, the air we breathe, and the soil in which we grow our food. Clearly, they are going to end up in our bodies as well.

Most of these toxins are acid forming or create acid by-products when our bodies attempt to filter them. What's more, they are often stored in fat in our bodies as a way to keep them out of our bloodstream, where they can do more damage.

We are often our own worst enemies when it comes to toxic exposure. Despite the attractive names, appealing fragrances, and slick advertising of so-called natural ingredients, many laundry and personal care products as well as household cleaning products contain some of the worst toxic compounds. These products include most commercially branded:

- Laundry detergents
- Fabric softeners
- Room deodorizers and air fresheners
- Perfumes and colognes
- Deodorants
- Shampoos, conditioners, and hair sprays
- Cosmetics

While I detail the many health hazards of these toxins in my books *The Brain Wash* and *The 4-Week Ultimate Body Detox Plan*, you need to know that the majority of these toxins will also acidify your body and be stored in fat. Now you might want to reconsider buying that perfume, fabric softener, or scented candle. Most health food stores have a wide array of natural personal care products, laundry and cleaning products, air fresheners, and other items that don't contain the same toxic ingredients as most commercial products. Be sure to read labels.

Acidity and Infections

In our everyday lives, we are all exposed to countless microbes—bacteria, fungi, viruses, yeasts, mold, and amoebas—that can be helpful, harmless, or dangerous. In fact, many germs live in our bodies, and an acidic environment provides them with an ideal opportunity to thrive. Not only do these germs live inside us 24/7, but we also have to contend with the acidic waste and by-products that some of them create as a result of their metabolic processes. Many researchers have identified overacidification of our body tissues and fluids as a precursor to microbial infections. If we keep our bodies close to an alkaline state, we make it very difficult for harmful germs to survive. Greater acidity increases vulnerability to these infections. Conversely, a healthy microbial balance creates conditions where it is easier to become and stay alkaline.

One of the best examples occurs during the holiday season. Imagine you have attended three social events over the weekend: a work party on Friday night, a gathering with friends on Saturday evening, and a family brunch on Sunday morning. Early in the following workweek, you are feeling exhausted and achy and suspect you have a fever. The common reaction is to assume you picked up a bug from someone you were exposed to at one of the parties. But chances are the extra sugar in the holiday treats and alcohol suppressed your immune system for 4 to 6 hours and acidified your body, giving that bug a chance to take hold and proliferate. It doesn't take much sugar to have this kind of result—even a few tea-spoons—and by the time the negative effects of the first pastry and glass of wine are wearing off, you have a craving for Aunt Emma's cherry pie and a glass of punch, not because they are tasty (even if they are) but because of the blood sugar fluctuations caused by the first hit of sugar. It's easy to blame the guy who was blowing his nose at the office party, but what's the likelihood that you overindulged in acidic sweets or other acidic foods during the holidays? We eat so many acid-forming foods, even when we are consciously trying to eat healthy, that chances are we have sabotaged ourselves during the festive season.

The Danger of the Acidic Diet

Without a doubt, the single greatest threat to our pH balance is an acidic diet. We have to eat every day, multiple times a day, so eliminating food is not an option—nor should it be. The goal is to eliminate the acidic foods all too common in our diets. Sweets, meat, dairy, trans fats, chemical additives, white flour and sugar, and fried foods all make it impossible to maintain or restore balance. The damage is cumulative as our glands, tissues, and organs deal with a chronic acid overload over the course of our life. Most acidic foods that find their way into our diets lack the vitamins, minerals, fiber, enzymes, and other nutritional elements that work with our body to restore balance and heal the existing damage our way of eating has caused. The absence of nutritional, pH-balancing food further exacerbates our overwhelmed, acidic bodies.

Chronic Acidity and Your Long-Term Health

Scientific research into human physiology has illustrated that healthy humans have built-in mechanisms that maintain blood pH within a very narrow range. Some researchers believe that these mechanisms are ade-quate to combat acidity and that an acidic diet could not alter blood pH in any measurable way. These scientists believe that the body always maintains a 7.365 pH and that acid-alkaline balance doesn't shift one way or another. They also suggest that eating an acid-forming diet has no effect on blood or tissue pH because the body always restores balance.

I agree with the traditional medical belief that the body uses its amazing innate intelligence to restore balance. The way it maintains body temperature provides a useful example. The human body needs to maintain a fairly narrow temperature range, ideally around 98.6°F. If body temperature drops a little lower, we start shivering in an effort to increase our temperature. A fairly small increase above 98.6°F is evidence of a fever, and the body induces sweating in an effort to reduce body temperature.

The human body strives continuously for a healthy biochemical balance as well. It activates processes to maintain homeostasis (or balance), such as breathing, blood circulation, digestion, and hormone production. In addition to these basic life functions, the body has other mechanisms for restoring pH balance when it is shifting too far to the acid side of the spectrum. The kidneys, for example, are detoxification organs designed to excrete acid to help us keep the balance required for the proper function- ing of our cells and systems. Other processes in our body dump alkaline minerals into the blood to neutralize its acidity.

Recent research has provided credible evidence that the modern diet is not only full of acid-forming foods, but that it is also disrupting our acid-base metabolism in ways our bodies were never intended to address. The human body and its acid-controlling processes were designed to manage and correct minor variations in pH. At no time in our evolution as a species have humans consumed such large amounts of meat, dairy, and sugar. Our bodies were never intended to process carbonated beverages, food additives and colors, and unhealthy fats. These items fall outside the body's directions for use. Add the strain of our chronically stressful lives and you can understand how quickly our bodies become overwhelmed and unable to manage the toxic load.

This constant battle waged by your cells and organs to regulate your body's pH takes its toll, leading to health problems and disease. Disease can be either the direct result of acidity or the result of your body's inability to keep up with the acid load it faces. Either way, you are left with strained organs and systems and depleted mineral reserves.

Signs of Chronic Acidity

Of course, carrying excess weight is one of the surest signs that your body has been chronically acidic for some time. But there are other signs of an acid-alkaline imbalance. They include pain, headaches, skin problems, frequent colds or flu, sinus infections, breathing troubles, allergies, inflammation, bloating, digestive disturbances or indigestion, muscle cramps, and perhaps the most common one, fatigue.

Most people find that their symptoms start out gradually and worsen over time. Eventually, glands and organs can be impacted by the excess acid. Usually the first organs to experience the effects of excess acidity are the thyroid glands (butterfly-shaped glands at the front of your neck), the adrenal glands (two triangular organs in the solar plexus region of the abdomen), and the liver. I've included information later in this book to help you assess whether you may be experiencing imbalances in the thyroid, adrenals, or liver. And, of course, I'll offer suggestions on how to address these imbalances and fine-tune the 60 Seconds to Slim program to best suit your individual needs.

Other problems can ensue when your pH is chronically acidic. That's because the acidity causes a reduction in oxygen levels, which can cause cells to die. With reduced oxygen and cellular destruction, any number of health issues can arise, including allergies, asthma, arthritis, or cancer, among others. So what often happens when people follow the 60 Seconds to Slim program is that they lose weight and frequently see improvements in their overall health too. That's not a bad side effect, is it?

Acidity and Metabolism

In addition to a balanced pH, proper metabolism depends on sufficient enzymes and coenzymes. Enzymes are special types of proteins that consist of long amino acid chains. They act as catalysts for every biochemical process in your body. There are thousands of different types of enzymes, with each kind serving a specific purpose of metabolism. In other words, enzyme A cannot do the job of enzyme Q. Enzymes are critical to our health and every biochemical process in our bodies. Without them, we could not live.

Enzymes are classified into three main types based on where they are found: metabolic enzymes (found in the body), food enzymes (you guessed it, found in food), and digestive enzymes (found specifically in the digestive tract). There is some overlap, as enzymes found in food aid digestion.

So why are we talking about enzymes in a book about balancing your body chemistry for weight loss? Healthy weight depends on the proper functioning of metabolic and digestive enzymes, as well as enzymes ingested from food. But enzymes can only work under the right conditions. One of the conditions is the correct pH balance, so we've started addressing this issue. Additionally, acidity in the body or in the diet can damage enzymes needed for healthy metabolism. So healthy body chemistry is integrally linked to healthy enzyme functions, which is integrally linked to healthy metabolism and weight balance.

Yet most of us don't have enough enzymes to maintain strong digestion and weight balance. Here are some reasons why:

1. Chronic stress depletes enzymes or the nutrients they need to work properly.
2. Drinking water, juice, soda, or other beverages with meals dilutes enzymes, making them less effective.
3. Cooking, canning, microwaving, baking, and broiling all reduce the enzymes in food, and many packaged foods have denatured during processing.
4. Insufficient chewing can put a strain on our body's ability to manufacture the enzymes needed to digest the specific type of foods we're eating, such as proteins, carbs, and fats.
5. Insufficient chewing also fails to release the enzymes present in any raw foods.
6. Eating too much of a particular type of food, such as carbohydrates, puts a strain on the body's ability to manufacture the enzymes needed to digest this type of food—a common problem for many overweight individuals.
7. We may have impaired organ function, including reduced pancreatic or liver function due to genetics or health issues.
8. Taking antacids with meals disrupts the pH balance in the stomach, causing food to be released into the intestines too quickly, before the stomach can adequately digest it.

9. We may make unhealthy dietary and lifestyle choices such as drinking alcohol, overeating, smoking, overusing medications, or eating foods containing artificial flavors and colors.

Enzymes work as catalysts to allow specific biochemical processes to occur. All three types of enzymes play a role in achieving or maintaining a healthy weight. Let's explore each type now.

METABOLIC ENZYMES

Your body manufactures metabolic enzymes to ensure the proper functioning of every process within it, from moving to breathing. Maintaining a healthy weight depends on many enzymes working smoothly in your body. A deficiency in any particular metabolic enzyme can have disastrous consequences for your health. We won't be getting into too much detail about these enzymes. For now, it is critical to understand that if your body doesn't produce adequate digestive enzymes (which we'll discuss momentarily), the liver and pancreas shift their focus from metabolic enzymes for vital life functions to digestion. So improving the functioning of our digestive enzymes takes the burden off the liver and pancreas. Both of these organs have essential roles to play in weight loss and maintaining a healthy weight, such as burning fat for energy, so relieving their digestive roles can help.

Since I'll be using the word *metabolism* a fair bit and we hear about it in the media, let me clarify what I mean by it. Metabolism is the process of converting the food we ingest into the energy we need for our bodies to function properly. This is a series of biochemical processes that nourishes our cells and keeps us alive. There are two types of metabolism: anabolism and catabolism. Anabolism refers to the cells' use of energy to perform life functions, including building complex molecules and cell structures. Catabolism refers to the breakdown of complex molecules to release energy.

Metabolism is a complex set of reactions that creates heat, carbon dioxide, water, and waste products. Much of the waste that is produced comes from acidic foods or drinks we've ingested. You may have heard the computer science acronym GIGO, which means "garbage in, garbage out." That concept is especially relevant to metabolism. If you ingest processed food full of chemicals and additives, your body simply cannot metabolize it properly, so it creates a lot of acidic waste. We have to reduce the waste—and the acid—so it cannot do damage to the body.

FOOD ENZYMES

I already stated that food enzymes, sometimes called plant enzymes, are found in food. But they are not found in just any food: Raw, unprocessed fruits, vegetables, nuts, seeds, and herbs contain enzymes. While meat and some other foods may contain enzymes in their raw state as well, eating raw meat can be dangerous. So I'm not including meat and poultry when I refer to raw foods. When food has been heated to over 118°F, its enzymes are destroyed. That includes almost all packaged and processed foods, all foods found in cans or jars, and baked, broiled, boiled, microwaved, barbecued, or otherwise cooked foods.

On the 60 Seconds to Slim program, vegetables are our primary source of enzymes, followed by nuts, seeds, fruit, and herbs. These ingredients are combined deliciously in the 60 Seconds to Slim recipes to make healing meals you will love.

DIGESTIVE ENZYMES

Strong digestion is critical to healthy metabolism and balanced weight. Actually, it's critical to great health in general. Enzymes are largely responsible for digestive processes working smoothly. In my experience, I've found that most overweight people have weak digestive systems and depleted enzyme stores. Improving the strength of your digestive system is one of the goals of *60 Seconds to Slim.*

Many different digestive enzymes are found in your body. These are also sometimes called pancreatic enzymes because they are secreted mostly by the pancreas. The pancreas is a thin organ that sits under the lower left side of your rib cage. It regulates blood sugar through the production and secretion of insulin. It also manufactures and secretes over 20 enzymes essential to digestion, the most common being amylase, lipase, and protease enzymes. These hardworking enzymes digest carbohydrates, fats, and proteins, respectively.

Protease enzymes work by breaking down protein molecules in your food into smaller molecules known as amino acids, which can be absorbed through the walls of the intestines, where they then become the building blocks for hormones, organs, and tissues. Without these enzymes, you would lack the amino acids necessary for your body to function properly. You might suffer from a hormonal imbalance that leads to weight gain or depression, or another serious health concern.

When we eat the Standard American Diet, which is almost devoid of enzymes, we rely heavily on our body to manufacture them. Over time, we can deplete our body's energy and capacity to manufacture sufficient enzymes. That's why so many of us could eat anything when we were kids but have bloating, indigestion, or other digestive symptoms when we eat the same foods now—our body can't keep up with the demand for digestive enzymes.

Don't believe claims that certain foods can travel through your digestive tract without being digested, and therefore have no calories and lead to weight loss. This is a slick marketing claim with no basis in human physiology. Your body will attempt to digest everything you put into your mouth and expend its digestive enzymes to break down larger molecules into smaller and smaller ones. Even if the food is not digestible, your body will waste its precious energy and enzymes attempting to digest it. In other words, stay away from these "fake foods" or "plastic foods," as I like to call them. They are simply not food as nature intended it.

The reality is that the strength of your digestion plays a significant role in determining your health and weight. Eating foods that balance your body chemistry, contain enzymes, or support your enzyme health helps you to restore balanced weight and better overall health.

As I mentioned earlier, enzyme activity is influenced by the pH of the body. We need to maintain a healthy pH level so our enzymes work effectively. By balancing our pH, we will start to have additional benefits from improving our body's enzyme activity. Enzyme function can also be impacted by drugs and toxins, both of which can interfere with enzymes and shift the acid-base balance in favor of acidity. Additionally, when the body uses minerals such as calcium and magnesium to nullify excessive amounts of acid, we may have insufficient amounts of these minerals left for other functions, including ensuring our enzymes are working properly. Let's explore how acid interacts with some important minerals in our body.

Assimilating Minerals

Chronic acidity can interfere with our body's ability to absorb, transport, and use minerals for their many functions. Some minerals need a small pH range to be assimilated. Take iodine, for instance. This essential mineral is needed for proper thyroid function, yet it requires an almost perfect pH balance for our thyroid to use it. The thyroid glands, the butterfly-shaped glands in the throat, are critical to establishing a healthy, balanced weight and ensuring a strong, fat-burning metabolism. Without sufficient iodine, they simply will not work well.

Calcium and potassium do not require such pH perfection and can be absorbed in the body in a wider pH range. Magnesium and sodium have an even greater pH range for absorption. Minerals such as iron, manganese, copper, and zinc fall somewhere between iodine and calcium in terms of the optimum pH range for absorption. But all of these minerals are essential to health. A deficiency in a single nutrient due to excess acidity or insufficient dietary intake can throw off a whole range of functions and lead to further imbalanced weight and poor health.

The Realities of Aging

While our bodies often become less effective with wear and tear, it isn't a necessary part of aging. Our acidic diet and lifestyle can weaken detoxification organs, bones, and muscles, further compromising our ability to cope with acidity. The Standard American Diet simply exacerbates this problem. By burdening our bodily systems with excess acid on an ongoing basis, we increase the likelihood of gaining weight or suffering from illness. The good news is that the acidity can be reversed. And if you're like many people, doing so may actually make you feel like you're reversing the effects of aging too.

Coping with Acid

The body has many mechanisms to ensure a healthy acid-alkaline balance. They are categorized as two main processes: (1) The body tries to expel excess acid through its various detoxification organs (filtering acid via the kidneys or exhaling acidic gases from the lungs are two of the main ones), and (2) it neutralizes acid waste with alkaline substances, of which there are many, including the minerals calcium and magnesium. These minerals are derived from the diet and stored in our body in the bones, muscles, and other tissues.

Your body's first acid-balancing mechanism is to attempt to eliminate acidity. One of the body's initial lines of defense against acid is the kidneys. The kidneys will attempt to dump excess acid in the urine so it is quickly eliminated.

Your Kidneys

Your kidneys are two small organs in the solar plexus region of your abdomen. They perform many valuable functions essential to life. Some of the main ones include filtering the blood and providing it with beneficial sugars, water, and amino acids that the body can use for its many functions; striving to maintain balance in your body, especially mineral, fluid, and pH balance; excreting toxins (including excess acid); and regulating blood pressure through hormone production.

You may be wondering where all these toxins come from. They can find their way into the body through chemicals, additives, or acid waste from metabolizing the food we eat and the beverages we drink. They can be created by the body as normal by-products of metabolism, or our bodies can excrete excess stress hormones due to a chronically stressful life and our inability to manage stress. Or toxins may be the by-product of the body's attempts to kill viruses, fungi, bacteria, or other pathogens that try to call it home.

No matter where the toxins originate, they share some common characteristics: (1) They can upset the natural balance of the body and clog its processes if they are not filtered out, and (2) the vast majority of toxins are acidic and can create a buildup of acidity if they remain in the body. So, while other organs and organ systems are involved with detoxification, the kidneys are doubly important when it comes to balancing pH, thanks to their ability to eliminate acid wastes.

When we eat high-protein foods like meat, the body breaks down the protein into its foundational elements, in this case, amino acids. Amino acids, or aminos, as they are often called, are critical to your body since they are needed to build all types of healthy tissue. However, during the metabolism of foods containing protein—particularly animal protein— urea, an acid by-product, is formed and can build up in the body if you are eating too much protein for your kidneys to handle. Some diet programs actually attempt to create such a situation, but it can be harmful in the long term (and sometimes even in the short term), depending on the acid levels in your body. This is why I encourage people to stay away from high-protein fad diets: They create acid buildup and put a strain on the kidneys. Additionally, most people think excess carbs will create fat stores in the body, but they aren't aware that excess protein has the same effect!

So if your kidneys cannot remove the excess urea and therefore are incapable of removing other acids and toxins from the blood, these acids and toxins may accumulate in the tissues, resulting in inflammation, weight gain, and even pain.

I'll be discussing ways to eliminate toxic waste from the body throughout *60 Seconds to Slim*, but for now, here are three easy ways to help your kidneys eliminate these toxins: (1) Drink more water to help the kidneys flush them; (2) eat fewer acid-forming foods (I'll explain more momentarily, but in general, reduce the amount of sugar, dairy, meat, and poultry in your diet); and (3) eat more alkalizing food (I'll go into greater detail later but the main thing is to start eating more nonstarchy vegetables).

Consider a typical meal for most people. It might be a burger or two (or maybe more) on buns made from white flour, accompanied by fries, soda, and some cookies. Or it could be a steak dinner with mashed potatoes, a white flour dinner roll (or two or more), coffee, and a piece of pie. Everything in both of these meals has an acid-forming effect on the body. Your kidneys must excrete all the acid by-products of attempting to digest the meat, potatoes, soda, coffee, and desserts. As you are learning in this chapter, the whole body suffers as it tries to remove excess acid. The result? As individuals and as a society, we are dealing with the ravages of chronic acidity in the form of unprecedented amounts of excess weight, obesity, heart disease, diabetes, cancer, and other health issues.

Perhaps part of the problem is that we don't see an immediate cause and effect. As a society, we are conditioned to expect things immediately. That's part of the popularity of fast food—it shows up almost as soon as you ask for it. So we think the same thing is true of cause and effect. If we don't see the effects of our lifestyle choices immediately, then they must not be relevant. But the effects of acidic buildup rarely show up right away. More likely, chronic acidity slowly breaks down normal processes in the body and gradually causes weight gain.

Acid-forming foods such as meat, dairy products, sugary sweets, coffee, tea, soda, and other items are called acidic because they leave a net acid load in your body. By that I mean that after these foods are metabolized by your body and burned for fuel, the residue they leave causes your tissues and bodily fluids to be more acidic than before you ate them. Keep in mind that I'm not talking about heartburn, although you may experience that as well. When almost every meal—or perhaps every meal—is acid forming, like the Standard American Diet, it can leave us in a chronic state of acidity. A few leafy greens or vegetables simply can't overcome the overwhelming amount of acid from the rest of our diet.

Consider the following meal: a turkey sandwich on whole wheat bread with a slice or two of tomato and a few leafy greens, topped with mustard and mayonnaise, and washed down with apple juice. The turkey, whole wheat bread, mustard, mayonnaise, and apple juice are all acid forming, with only the few leafy greens and the tomato to balance them. As you can see, this causes a net acid load. You may be surprised to learn that raw tomatoes are alkalizing. Some foods, like tomatoes, lemons, limes, and grapefruits, may seem acidic, but they actually have an alkalizing effect on the body. I've provided a chart in the next chapter (see page 42) to help you learn which foods are acid forming and which are alkalizing.

Q&A Wise Acid Foods

Q: Are all the foods on the acid side of the 60 Seconds to Slim Acid-Alkaline Food Chart (see page 42) Wise Acid choices?

A: Not all foods on the acidic side of the table are Wise Acid foods. Some are unhealthy and are best avoided. Let's face it: Most of us know that a 16-ounce steak dinner with mashed potatoes followed by a large bowl of ice cream with chocolate sauce is not conducive to weight loss. Wise Acid foods include fresh fruit, raw nuts, whole grains, organic lean poultry and eggs (in moderation), fish, milk substitutes (like rice milk or organic soy milk), and some spices. Keep in mind that when I refer to fresh fruit, I'm not talking about canned fruit, which is not a Wise Acid food. In fact, it's not a health food at all.

I've listed common Wise Acid foods in the chart on pages 50–51, but it's impossible to list every food, so it's important to use your best judgment. Wise Acid foods are so named because they deliver so many health benefits. However, keep in mind that all acidic foods need to be balanced by lots of alkaline foods for best results.

Even many health-conscious eaters don't realize that their diet may still be highly acid forming. Fruits fall into a category of foods I call Wise Acid Foods, meaning they are acid forming but they have enough other merits to be included in moderation in your diet (see pages 50–51 for a chart of Wise Acid Foods). Yet the average health-conscious person tends to eat a fair amount of fruit, chooses whole grains (most of which are acid forming), and may eat lean chicken or fish (again, acid forming), along with vegetables, which are probably not consumed in sufficient quantities to offset the acid-forming foods.

I hope by now you're starting to get the picture that our diets, even some of the so-called healthy ones, are still acid forming and can cause us to become fat, fatigued, and unhealthy. We increase our risk of becoming overweight and of suffering long-term health problems by making food choices that strain our detoxifying organs, which attempt to filter the excess acid, and by depleting our stores of alkaline minerals in our bones and muscles, leaving them vulnerable as well.

THE KIDNEYS ATTEMPT TO NIX THE ACID

When our blood starts to become slightly acidic, the kidneys excrete ammonia into the urine, causing a strong-smelling urine that can be an indicator that our body is becoming overly acidic. Urinary tract infections can result from the excess acid buildup, preventing the kidneys from managing their workload. Bladder or kidney infections can also be a sign that the acid waste hasn't been sufficiently removed because the kidneys cannot handle the excessive acid buildup. Kidney stones may also form because of the acid waste buildup. These are some of the signs that the body is overly acidic and some of its first lines of defense cannot keep pace with their load.

The Lungs Get Involved

While the kidneys are the key players in the fight to detoxify acidity, the lungs are also involved. They remove carbon dioxide as a way to maintain acid-alkaline balance and to ensure proper respiration. Deep breathing, which few of us do, increases the level of oxygen in our blood, thereby helping the body to remove acid wastes through the exhalation of carbon dioxide. That's why deep-breathing techniques and exercises that encourage them, such as yoga, qigong, and moderate aerobic exercise, can be helpful. Keep in mind that excessive exercise creates a buildup of lactic acid, and you can probably guess from the name that the result is more acid, so it's wise to avoid overdoing it. However, that's not an issue for most of us who rarely pick ourselves up off the couch, so please don't use it as an excuse to avoid exercising. Your body needs to move, and it needs the deep breathing that comes along with it.

Other Detox Organs

The kidneys and lungs are supported in their acid-eliminating roles by other organs including the liver, the intestines, and the skin. The liver filters toxic substances that are typically acid forming. The intestines expel acid by excreting it in our bowel movements. And some acid is eliminated through sweat when we perspire.

Acid: Neutralized

So now you understand how the body tries to filter excess acid by excreting it via the kidneys, lungs, liver, intestines, and skin. But, as mentioned, filtering is not the only way the body attempts to cope with acid. There are also storehouses of alkaline minerals and other nutrients and substances that the body uses as a type of alkaline bank, including calcium, magnesium, potassium, bicarbonate, and the amino acid glutamine. These stores are primarily found in the bones and the muscles.

THEM BONES, THEM ALKALINE BONES

As most of you are aware, bones are rich in calcium. That's why so many people pop calcium tablets to help build their bones. What most people don't realize is that the bones act like bank accounts for calcium and that the calcium doesn't just enter the bones when we ingest it or take supplements with it. Instead, calcium deposits and withdrawals are regularly made. Our bones are heavily involved with maintaining pH balance in our bodies. After your body becomes excessively acidic and your detox organs (like the kidneys) have attempted to eliminate the acid, if there is still acid remaining, then your bones will dump calcium into the blood to help restore acid-alkaline balance. Calcium does this by creating oxygen at the cellular level, which creates a more alkaline body. The body is immensely wise and knows that the acidity can have disastrous consequences, so it will sacrifice minerals from the bones to prevent acidic blood and other bodily fluids from wreaking havoc on your organs and organ systems, particularly the brain. The blood's pH must be maintained at 7.365, so the body takes what might seem like drastic measures to ensure it is balanced.

While it may sound odd that the body would sacrifice calcium from the bones to restore pH levels of blood and other bodily fluids, let's explore a bit of background about calcium in the body to help you to further understand why this happens.

Calcium is found in high amounts in the body, more so than many other minerals. That's because it is arguably involved in more functions in the body than other minerals. Calcium helps to regulate our heartbeat, cellular function, bone health, and muscle movement, among many other functions.

Does that mean you should just pop more calcium tablets to solve your pH imbalance? Unfortunately, it does not. While calcium is found in everything from heartburn tablets to dairy products to coral calcium and other mineral supplements, that doesn't mean that all of these sources are beneficial, nor does it mean that they will all help balance your body chemistry. While calcium supplement manufacturers regularly attempt to degrade vegetables as sources of calcium, the reality is that vegetables are the best sources with proven benefits. Calcium supplements, meanwhile, are often adulterated through chemical processing or contaminated by lead.

While calcium dumping from the bones is a valid short-term solution to rebalance the body's biochemistry, the problem lies in continuously eating acidic foods and beverages and living a highly stressful (read: acid-forming) lifestyle. Over time, the bones can become depleted because of their calcium-sacrificing tendencies.

There are a few other issues with regard to calcium in our bodies. Most of us don't eat enough biologically active calcium—calcium that our bodies can use effectively to benefit our health. Biologically active calcium is primarily found in leafy green vegetables, seeds, nuts, and legumes. Even when we do get enough calcium from those sources, we also eat excessive acidic foods that force our bodies to deplete stored calcium as described above. Additionally, dairy products, the primary sources of calcium in our diet, are acid forming, thereby increasing our calcium requirement.

A study by David Bushinsky, MD, professor of medicine at the University of Rochester Medical Center, provides proof that we lose critical calcium alongside acid in our urine. His research showed that chronic acidity caused calcium excretion in urine; however, no change in intestinal calcium absorption was observed. We absorb most nutrients, including calcium, through the walls of our intestines. The study also showed that bone is a reservoir for potassium and sodium, and that bone receptor sites that normally bind with these minerals, as well as hydrogen, cannot function properly when the body is excessively acidic. In that case, the hydrogen bumps potassium and sodium off the surface of the bone to buffer the acid, further depleting the bones of minerals critical for their health.[3]

When there is a net loss of calcium (more is withdrawn from the bones than deposited), it is rarely restored by eating the Standard American Diet, even with supplements. It is essential to address the source of the problem—excess acidity—to adequately address bone demineralization.

THE MUSCLES AND PH

The muscles also play a role in neutralizing excessive acid. They store nutrients like magnesium and glutamine which is an amino acid, a building block of protein foods. When the blood pH becomes slightly acidic, glutamine is released from skeletal muscle to restore balance. While the blood becomes balanced, giving up glutamine causes a loss of muscle protein, which can result in muscle weakness. Glutamine is found in fish, red meat, beans, and dairy products, most of which are acid forming, but I'll discuss solutions for this later in the book. It reduces acidity by binding hydrogen ions (electrically charged cells) to form ammonium (alkaline) in a process called *nitrogen fixation*. Like calcium dumped from the bones, glutamine is sacrificed to neutralize acid. And the release of this nutrient results in muscle loss in the same way that the use of calcium for neutralizing acid causes bone density loss.

The muscles also dump the mineral magnesium, since it is alkaline, to help neutralize excess acid. Like calcium, magnesium is essential for many critical body functions. It is required for a healthy heart and healthy muscles, nerves, hormones, blood vessels, and teeth and even balances moods. It activates around 500 enzymes in your body that themselves are essential for many functions, including those involved in insulin secretion and the body's use of sugar. Insulin is the hormone secreted by your pancreas to help balance blood sugar, remember, but it signals your body to store fat, so ensuring that insulin is properly secreted requires sufficient magnesium and the enzymes it coaxes. We'll be discussing this topic more in-depth later in the book.

Balancing Weight and Health

I think you get the picture: Our bodies always strive for balance but they can only do so much if they are fed denatured, nutrient-deprived foods. And when they are out of balance, bones may become depleted, muscles weakened, kidneys taxed, lungs overburdened, and on and on.

Our bodies have many innate pH-balancing or neutralizing mechanisms to ensure our blood never deviates too far from its ideal place of 7.365 on the pH spectrum. It is mind-boggling to think of just how miraculous our bodies are. They juggle trillions of functions every single second. But it is incorrect to think that our bodies can simply go on endlessly balancing our blood, or other bodily fluids, or tissue pH levels without significant consequences when they are fed nutritionally inferior, acid-forming food. Our diets just don't have enough calcium or magnesium to manage the ongoing mineral dumping from our bones and muscles. According to some experts, 79 percent of Americans are deficient in calcium and 67 percent are deficient in magnesium. Plus, our acid-forming diets increase our need for these minerals.

Currently, the medical community measures the acid-alkaline balance only when things get out of control and enter life-threatening territory, in the form of chronic metabolic or respiratory acidosis. But what about the wear-and-tear effects of acid on an ongoing basis and its ability to overwhelm organs and deplete mineral and amino acid stores? Our bodies develop coping mechanisms, and weight gain is one of the main ones that indicates we have overwhelmed their capacities to deal with an ongoing onslaught of acidic foods and beverages. The acid gets buffered by fat stores. A blood test may not accurately reflect the level of acidity because the acid is not running through our bloodstream; instead, it is conveniently packed away on our thighs, abdomen, buttocks, or other fatty areas. So a normal blood test may not reflect how your pH levels are chronically out of balance. Our bodies have found a way to buffer the acid by making us fat.

The good news is that our diets are so acid forming that it is easy to make them more alkaline. Studies show, however, that even when a diet has been changed to become more alkaline, acid excretion continues. That might sound like a bad thing—but it's not. It means that your body is trying to eliminate the acid buildup in your fat and your organs are more capable of displacing the acid from your body. So while *60 Seconds to Slim* is designed for 4 weeks, you may find that it is a lifestyle you want to continue. After all, people experience a variety of positive side effects, including pain reduction, increased energy, improved mobility, and an overall sense of vitality.

Chapter 2

Fire Up Your Metabolism

Getting Started on The Essential Plan

Now that you have an understanding of the importance of balancing your body chemistry, I'll share the fundamentals of the 60 Seconds to Slim Plan so you can get started balancing your pH and losing weight. This chapter provides the first layer of lifestyle and dietary advice you will follow over the next 4 weeks—or for as long as you need in order to reach your weight-loss goal. When you are ready to maintain your healthy weight, this is also the plan you will rely on to stay slim and hold on to your revitalized health for life.

I call it The Essential Plan, and it is the basis of your alkalizing strategy. When you feel comfortable with the information presented in this chapter and you've started making the recommended changes to your diet and lifestyle, you can start to add the 60-Second Weight-Loss Tips that begin in the next chapter.

Keep in mind that we'll be exploring different foods and strategies in greater detail as we progress. I'll be explaining the research and rationale behind each part of the plan throughout this chapter, so don't worry if you're feeling confused. It will all make sense by the end of this chapter!

Note: While the 60 Seconds to Slim Plan is designed to be implemented over 4 weeks (jumping into Week 1 at the same time as The Essential Plan), it's okay to spend a week or more just living by The Essential Plan to get used to these guidelines before starting Week 1. You can also spend additional weeks adjusting to each new phase. In this way, you can customize the plan to your particular needs and your preferred pace, which will help you make changes that last.

Kick Acid to Lose Weight and Boost Energy

In the last chapter you learned that too much acid in your body can cause weight gain, fatigue, inflammation, pain, and a host of other health problems. Later in this chapter, you will learn about many of the acid-forming foods that tip your pH out of balance. But before we get to the foods you'll need to eat less of, I want to go over the alkalizing foods that are essential to getting your weight and health back on track.

First, let's revisit the pH scale. As you learned earlier, the pH scale measures the level of acidity or alkalinity. Just as you don't need to be a biochemist to understand the pH scale, you don't need a PhD in chemistry to alkalize your body. Remember that the pH scale is like a tug-of-war in your body. On one side is the acid team and on the other side is the alkaline team. The middle is neutral. Most of what we eat and most of our lifestyle choices tip the balance in favor of acidity. However, your blood needs to remain stable at 7.365 (slightly alkaline) to maintain health and life. We cannot live if our body becomes too acidic, so the body has mechanisms in place to ensure that the blood, which feeds our brain and all our organs, glands, and tissues, remains slightly alkaline. One of the ways the body deals with acidity is to store it in fat cells as a way to get it out of the blood quickly. Fat cells are your body's natural buffer against acid since they have a natural affinity for acidic toxins. Fat is actually your body's ally against acidic food choices. Kicking acid out of your diet gives your body a chance to restore balance at the cellular level, which allows it to start breaking down fat stores and ultimately to rebalance your weight.

Acidity can also impair the proper functioning of our hormonal systems, sap our energy, and leave us prone to illness and pain. It impairs many of our organs' abilities to keep us slim and healthy. However, kicking out harmful acidic foods is insufficient. You also need to add more alkalizing foods and water to ensure that your body gets back on track and to maximize fat burning.

Next let's explore the many alkalizing food options to help you balance your pH and lose weight.

Foods That Alkalize Your Body

I am regularly asked which foods are acidic and which ones are alkaline. So I've created a handy chart of more than 200 foods to help you discern between those that are acid-forming and those that are alkalizing over the coming weeks or months, making it easier for you to eat a more alkalizing diet. Don't worry about memorizing it. Make a copy and put it on your fridge. Carry a copy in your purse or somewhere you'll have it when you head to the grocery store. It won't be long before you have a strong handle on which foods are acidic and which ones are alkaline.

You may be surprised to see that most fruits are acidic. This is the nutrition news that shocks people the most. When I first started out in the natural health field over two decades ago, I learned that fruits, while acidic, become alkaline in your body after you eat them. Well, that's true of lemons, limes, and tart cherries, but the sugar content in most fruits overrides the minerals and other substances that would normally help a food to be alkaline. So you can eat fruits (as I'll discuss in greater detail momentarily), but it's best to focus on avocados, tomatoes, unsweetened coconut, grapefruits, lemons, and limes. Also note that tomatoes, when cooked, become slightly acidic, but they are slightly alkaline when raw. Other than that, fruits are a Wise Acid food. Wise Acids have many healthful nutrients and phytonutrients but should still be eaten sparingly when you're trying to lose weight. The sugar content can cause wild blood sugar fluctuations that lead to fat storage, and that's not something we want.

7 Easy Ways to Alkalize Yourself

Kick acid by making 70 percent of your diet alkaline foods. Some excellent alkalizing options:

1. **Eat more veggies.** Most vegetables are alkalizing to your body. So eat your salad greens, beets, broccoli, celery, carrots, cucumbers, peppers, onions, garlic, spinach, sweet potatoes, and yams.

2. **Select great grains.** Whole grains like quinoa, spelt, buckwheat groats, and millet are alkalizing. While there are many otherwise healthy whole grain options, many are acid forming.

3. **Drink lots of purified water.** Add pH drops, green powder, or fresh lemon juice and drink the mixture 20 minutes before meals for optimum results.

4. **Choose almond or coconut milk over dairy products.** These are readily available in most supermarkets and health food stores and are delicious as substitutions in baked goods or on their own.

5. **Enjoy alkaline fruits.** These include avocado, sour cherries, fresh coconut, grapefruit, tomatoes (cooked tomatoes are mildly acid forming), lemons, and limes. And while it is tempting to believe that all fruit is alkalizing to the body, keep in mind that it is just a myth, perpetuated by many well-intentioned people. Regardless, acid-forming fruits still have many health-boosting properties when eaten in moderation, which is why I consider them Wise Acid foods.

6. **Eat more beans, peas, and lentils.** For tasty recipe ideas, try cooking up Angela's Hearty Minestrone Soup (see page 256) or Roasted Red Pepper Hummus (see page 252).

7. **Try to eat a large salad daily.** Make the 60 Seconds to Slim Signature Salad (page 262) or Balsamic Salmon Spinach Salad (page 264). Choose a healthy dressing option like Asian Ginger Vinaigrette (page 271) or Greek Salad Dressing (page 269).

The Veggies Have It

Vegetables are among your best alkaline choices. Almost all vegetables are alkaline, unless they're overcooked or deep-fried. Potatoes are the exception—white, yellow, red, or purple potatoes are quite acid forming. Sweet potatoes, however, are alkalizing and can be easily incorporated into the 60 Seconds to Slim program.

I know you may be rolling your eyes at the thought of eating more vegetables, or any at all if you're currently eating the Standard American Diet. If you don't love vegetables, you simply haven't prepared them the right way. My husband was a vegetable-hater extraordinaire when we met. Now most of his favorite meals are vegetable dishes. The same could be true for you. So give the recipes in Part 3 a chance. Throughout *60 Seconds to Slim*, you'll find that your tastebuds will start to adapt and the flavors you once loved or craved no longer suit you. As your body becomes more biochemically balanced, your desire for healthy foods will shine through.

You can eat just about any type of vegetable you can find. But whatever you do, don't deep-fry it. Any of the alkalizing nutritional benefits of vegetables are lost when you add overheated, rancid, inflammatory oils like those used in deep-frying. Instead, sauté, pan-fry in olive or coconut oil, steam, stir-fry, bake, or roast vegetables. Or eat them raw by grating, mincing, or finely chopping them and adding them to salads, sandwiches, or wraps, or by having them as a stand-alone salad with dressing. A little creativity goes a long way toward making food you will love.

SALAD: IT'S NOT JUST ABOUT THE LEAVES

Forget boring salads made of nothing but tasteless iceberg lettuce and starchy tomatoes topped with some chemical-laced, disgusting bottled dressing. Salads on the 60 Seconds to Slim program are anything but boring. I love gourmet, hearty, meal-size salads full of delicious and nutritious ingredients. I encourage you to make them a regular part of your weight-loss efforts.

I frequently roast or sauté a few of my favorite foods like sweet potatoes and red peppers; or I caramelize some onions to top a large plate of greens. Add grated raw vegetables, a handful of berries, cooked chickpeas, fresh herbs, or some slices of avocado, and top with a homemade dressing. Enjoy this gourmet salad on its own or alongside some cooked wild salmon. Delish!

(continued on page 48)

The 60 Seconds to Slim

Acid-Alkaline Food Chart

Most Acidic	Moderately Acidic	Slightly Acidic	
Fruits			
All dried, pickled, or canned fruits	Apples Apricots Bananas Berries Cherries (sweet) Currants Figs (fresh) Grapes Guava Honeydew melon Mangos Oranges Papayas Peaches Pears Persimmons Pineapples Tangerines Watermelon	Cantaloupe Dates (fresh) Nectarines Plums	
Vegetables			

This chart will help you understand which foods are acidic and which ones are alkaline. If you print out the chart and put it on your fridge, you'll find you remember which ones are the best choices fairly quickly. Focus your efforts on the alkaline side of the chart; alkaline foods should make up 70 percent of your plate at every meal. It takes some time to develop new habits, but once you get used to making different foods or preparing the same foods in different ways, you'll soon see how delicious these foods can be and how great they'll make you feel.

Slightly Alkaline	Moderately Alkaline	Most Alkaline
Cherries (sour) Coconut Grapefruit Lemons Limes Tomatoes	Avocado	
Artichokes Asparagus Brussels sprouts	Arugula Beets Broccoli	Cucumbers Dandelion greens Kale

Most Acidic	Moderately Acidic	Slightly Acidic	

Vegetables *(cont.)*

Grains

Most Acidic	Moderately Acidic	Slightly Acidic	
Barley (pearl or pot) Corn Oat bran	Brown rice Oats Rye bread White bread Whole grain bread Wild rice	Amaranth Kasha Millet Triticale	

Legumes

		Black beans Chickpeas Kidney beans	

Nuts and Seeds

Cashews Peanuts Pistachios	Walnuts	Brazil nuts Flaxseeds Hazelnuts Pecans Sunflower seeds	

Slightly Alkaline	Moderately Alkaline	Most Alkaline
Carrots Cauliflower Chives Horseradish Kohlrabi Leeks Peas Rhubarb Rutabaga Sweet potatoes Turnips Watercress Yams Zucchini	Cabbage Celery Collard greens Endive Fresh ginger Garlic Green beans Mustard greens Okra Onions Peppers, bell Peppers, hot (fresh, not pickled) Radishes Salad greens Sorrel Spinach	Sea vegetables (such as agar, arame, dulse, hijiki, and nori) Sprouted beans (including soy spouts, mung bean sprouts) Sprouted seeds (alfalfa, red clover, and broccoli)
Buckwheat groats or flour Quinoa Spelt bread (yeast free, sugar free, and preservative free) Spelt grains or flour		
Lentils Soy flour Tofu	Edamame (green soybeans) Lima beans Navy beans	Soy lecithin Soy nuts
Almonds (raw, unsalted) Caraway seeds Cumin seeds Fennel seeds Sesame seeds		Pumpkin seeds

Most Acidic	Moderately Acidic	Slightly Acidic	
Oils and Fats			
	Butter Corn oil Margarine containing trans fats Trans fat–free margarine	Canola oil Grapeseed oil Sunflower oil Walnut oil	
Dairy Products and Milk Alternatives			
Casein Cheese (milk, goat, soy) Ice cream Whey Yogurt		Cow's milk Cream Rice milk Soy milk	
Meat, Fish, and Poultry			
Beef Eggs Fish, farmed Organ meats Pork Poultry Shellfish Veal	Fish, wild, ocean	Fish, wild, freshwater	
Spices, Condiments, and More			
Carob Cocoa Jam/Jelly Malt Mustard Rice syrup Soy sauce Vinegar	Ketchup Mayonnaise Nutmeg Table salt Vanilla	Curry powder	

Slightly Alkaline	Moderately Alkaline	Most Alkaline
Almond oil Avocado oil Borage oil Coconut oil Cod liver oil Evening primrose oil Flaxseed oil Olive oil Soy oil		
Almond milk (unsweetened) Coconut milk (unsweetened) Goat's milk		Human breast milk
	Fresh and dried herbs: basil, cilantro, oregano, parsley, rosemary, sage, thyme, etc. Ground red pepper	Celtic sea salt Himalayan crystal salt

SEA VEGETABLES

Sea vegetables are among the most nutritious foods on the planet. One of the richest sources of the thyroid-boosting mineral iodine, sea vegetables are easy to incorporate into your meals. Soak some finely sliced seaweed, like arame or wakame, in hot water for 5 minutes to rehydrate, drain, and throw on top of your favorite salad. Or wrap some cooked quinoa and cucumber or avocado slices in nori and enjoy a healthier take on sushi rolls.

SPROUTING A THINNER, HEALTHIER YOU

Sprouts are some of the healthiest, most alkalizing foods you can eat. That's because the nutritional count skyrockets when seeds are soaked and sprouted. The energy contained in the seed, grain, nut, or legume is ignited and its nutrients unlocked, providing a powerhouse of benefits. It always amazes me that so many lists of superfoods completely ignore the best superfoods of all—sprouts. And unlike expensive, exotic superfoods, sprouts are cheap and readily available. You can either purchase them from your local health food store or grocery store or grow them yourself. Growing your own sprouts is easier than you'd think—I provide instructions in 60-Second Weight-Loss Tip #33 (see page 151).

Whether you grow them yourself or purchase them, there are many reasons to consider adding sprouts to your diet. Here are seven:

1. Experts estimate that there can be up to 100 times more enzymes in sprouts than in uncooked fruits and vegetables. Enzymes are special types of proteins that act as catalysts for all your body's functions, including digestion and fat burning. By eating more enzyme-rich foods like sprouts, you not only take a load off of your enzyme-creating organs (like the pancreas, liver, salivary glands, and intestines), freeing up more energy for you, but you also ensure that you get the maximum nutritional value out of the food you eat. Extracting more vitamins, minerals, amino acids, essential fatty acids, and natural sugars (in moderation) from the foods you eat ensures that your entire body has the nutritional building blocks of life to help every one of its processes work more effectively.

2. During the soaking and sprouting process, the quality and the nutritional value of the protein in beans, nuts, seeds, and grains improves. The amino acid lysine, for example, which is needed to

prevent cold sores and to maintain a healthy immune system, increases significantly during the sprouting process.

3. The fiber content of beans, nuts, seeds, and grains increases substantially when they're sprouted. Fiber is critical to weight loss. It not only binds to fats and toxins in our body to escort them out, but it also ensures that any fat our body breaks down is moved quickly out of the body before it can resorb through the walls of the intestines (which is the main place for nutrient absorption into the blood).

4. Sprouting also dramatically increases vitamin content. This is especially true of vitamins A, C, and E and the B-complex vitamins. The vitamin content of some seeds, grains, beans, and nuts increases by up to 20 times within only a few days of sprouting. Research shows that during the sprouting process, mung bean sprouts (or just bean sprouts, as they are often called) increase in vitamin B_1 by up to 285 percent, vitamin B_2 by up to 515 percent, and niacin by up to 256 percent.

5. Essential fatty acids needed to break down fat in your body increase during the sprouting process. Most of us are deficient in these fat-burning essential fats because they are not common in our diet. Eating more sprouts is an excellent way to get more of these important nutrients.

6. During sprouting, minerals bind to protein in the seed, grain, nut, or bean, making them more usable in the body. This is true of alkaline minerals such as calcium and magnesium that help us to balance our body chemistry for weight loss and better health.

7. Sprouts are the ultimate locally grown food when you grow them yourself. You are helping the environment and ensuring that you are not getting unwanted pesticides, food additives, and other harmful fat-bolstering chemicals that thwart your weight-loss efforts.

Alkaline Fruits

Almost all fruits are acid forming. The exceptions are lemons, limes, grapefruit, fresh coconut, avocados, and tomatoes (unless the tomatoes are cooked, in which case they are slightly acid forming).

Enjoy fresh lemon or lime juice in your water to boost its alkalizing ability. Although these foods test acidic in a laboratory, they alkalize your

(continued on page 52)

Wise Acid Foods

"Dairy" Products	Meat, Poultry, and Fish	Legumes	Fruit	Grains
Rice milk, unsweetened Soy milk, unsweetened Vegan soy cheese (made without casein, sweeteners, preservatives, hydrogenated fats, or trans fats)	Beef, organic Eggs, organic Freshwater fish (wild only, not farmed) Ocean fish (wild only, not farmed) Organ meats, organic Poultry, organic	Black beans Chickpeas Kidney beans	All dried unsulphured fruit (in minimal amounts) Apples Apricots Bananas Berries Cantaloupe Cherries (sweet) Currants Dates (fresh) Figs (fresh) Grapes Guava Honeydew melon Mangos Nectarines Oranges Papaya Peaches Pears Persimmons Pineapple Plums Tangerines Watermelon	Amaranth Barley (pearl or pot) Brown rice Kasha Millet Oats Oat bran Organic corn (most non-organic corn is gentically modified and not recommended) Rye bread Triticale Wild rice

These acid-forming foods deliver many important nutrients and should comprise about 30 percent of your diet alongside lots of alkalizing foods.

Nuts and Seeds	Extras	Oils	Sweeteners	Beverages
Brazil nuts	Carob, organic, unsweetened	Butter	Cane juice	Black or green tea
Cashews, raw, unsalted	Cocoa, organic, unsweetened	Canola oil	Honey, unpasteurized	Fruit juice, unsweetened, with no preservatives, additives, or colors
Flaxseeds	Curry powder	Corn oil	Maple syrup	
Hazelnuts	Ketchup	Grape seed oil	Sugarcane, organic, unrefined	
Peanuts (only if they are extremely fresh since they are prone to toxic mold growth)	Mayonnaise	Margarine		
Pecans	Nutmeg	Sunflower oil		
Pistachios	Vanilla	Walnut oil		
Sunflower seeds				
Walnuts				

body to help balance your pH, burn fat, and boost health. Don't cook them, though—cooking can alter their health benefits. Enjoy fresh grapefruit for breakfast or as a snack or add wedges to your salads.

We typically think of avocados and tomatoes as vegetables, but they are actually fruits. Enjoy them raw in salads, salsa, guacamole, and more. Be sure to check out my recipes for Super Fat-Burning Salsa and Chunky Guacamole on pages 255 and 254. They're delicious! As noted above, cooking tomatoes turns them slightly acidic, but they still have many wonderful health properties worth keeping them in the 30 percent Wise Acid part of your diet.

You can also enjoy fresh coconut, unsweetened grated coconut, coconut juice, coconut milk, and coconut cream on their own or in recipes. I've included some excellent recipes that use coconut milk or cream in Part 3 of this book.

Since they are acidic, dried fruit such as raisins and prunes should be eaten sparingly. When you do indulge in these sweet snacks that are high in sugar, it's important to select dried fruits that are unsulphured.

Q&A Unsulphured Dried Fruit

Q. You mention that raisins and dried fruit should be unsulphured. What does that mean and how can I tell?

A: Most fruit is sprayed with either a sulphur or sugar solution prior to drying to prevent discoloration during the drying process. It's always best to choose unsulphured and unsweetened dried fruit. While the fruit may not look as vibrantly colored, it is more natural and better for your body.

Many health food stores and some grocery stores carry unsulphured dried fruit. The easiest way to tell if your fruit is unsulphured is to check the label. If you see *sulfites* or *sulphur* on the list, it's best to avoid those brands. You should also avoid sugar, which is often not listed on the label, making it difficult to determine whether fruit was coated in a sugar solution. If it is listed on the label it will be recognizable by the *-ose* ending, as in *glucose*, or may be listed as high fructose corn syrup. This is a clue that this particular fruit product is best avoided. Don't be deterred by unsulphured dried fruit that is a little brown compared with what you might be used to seeing. That's normal, and it is safe to eat.

The Whole Grain and Nothing but the Grain

Some of the best alkalizing grains include buckwheat groats or flour, quinoa, and spelt grains or flour. Quinoa and buckwheat are both gluten-free choices for people with gluten intolerance or sensitivity. Spelt is a whole grain that contains gluten but is fine for most people; try yeast-free, sugar-free, preservative-free spelt bread. If you haven't tried these grains, trust me, it's worth it. I've included some recipes for pancakes, flatbreads, and muffins made from these whole alkalizing grains. Also be sure to check out Tip #34 (page 158) to start reaping the benefits of fat-busting quinoa.

Legumes

There are many excellent alkalizing legumes and legume-based products, including soy lecithin, soy nuts, edamame (green soybeans), lima beans, navy beans, lentils, soy flour, and tofu. You can enjoy them in many different ways. I love lentils with onions and some curry spices or firm organic tofu cut into cubes and then marinated in a bit of gluten-free, preservative-free soy sauce or fresh lemon juice. After a day of marinating, it tastes like cheese but doesn't have the mucus-forming, acidifying effects of dairy. Or cook some navy beans and add cooked onions and tomato sauce for a delicious dish. There is an excellent recipe for Edamame Stir-Fry from my friend Dr. Cobi Slater on page 289.

Nuts and Seeds

While not all nuts and seeds are alkaline, many are. Enjoy them as snacks, as a vegetarian protein in your meals, or to benefit from their healthy fats, which give them the excellent ability to break down fats in your body. Enjoy raw unsalted pumpkin seeds, raw unsalted almonds, and sesame seeds, as well as some seeds used as spices, such as caraway, cumin, and fennel seeds. If you haven't tried cooked cabbage with cooked onions, cumin seeds, and some unrefined sea salt, you're missing out. I've served it to cabbage haters who loved it.

Oils

Many oils are alkalizing, including almond oil, avocado oil, borage oil, coconut oil, cod liver oil, evening primrose oil, flaxseed oil, olive oil, and soy oil. It's as important to purchase high-quality, cold-pressed oils from your local health food store as it is to cook the oils properly, if you cook them at all. Do not cook

(continued on page 56)

Create a Fat-Burning Gourmet
Salad
in Minutes

Bases (pick one or more)

Beetroot (grated)
Boston lettuce
Brown rice (cooked)
Endive
Grated cabbage
Leaf lettuce
Mixed greens (mesclun or spring mix)
Quinoa (cooked)
Radicchio
Romaine lettuce
Seaweed (such as arame, nori, or wakami)
Spinach
Watercress
Wild rice (cooked)

Mix-ins (pick three or more)

Alfalfa sprouts
Apples (sliced or grated)
Avocado
Bell peppers (red, green, or yellow)
Blackberries
Blueberries
Broccoli (finely chopped)
Broccoli sprouts
Carrots (julienned, roasted, or grated)
Celery
Celery root
Chickpeas
Cucumber slices
Edible flowers (such as nasturtiums, violas, or pansies)
Fenugreek sprouts
Grapefruit slices
Great Northern beans
Kidney beans
Lima beans
Mung bean sprouts
Mushrooms (raw or cooked)
Olives
Onion (minced)
Onion sprouts
Orange slices
Pea shoots
Peas (fresh)
Pinto beans
Pomegranate seeds
Radishes
Raspberries
Red clover sprouts
Scallions
Strawberries
Sweet potato (grated or roasted)
Tomatoes
Zucchini (grated or roasted)

I've included some excellent salad recipes in Part 3, but the best way to ensure that you eat a salad each day is to have fun experimenting with different combinations. Use this list for inspiration, and the possibilities will seem endless! Pick from each column below for a balanced, hearty salad, or make your own rules if you are feeling confident and creative.

Toppings (pick one or more)

Almond slices	Hazelnuts (chopped)
Carrots (grated)	Herbs (such as thyme, oregano, and garlic, minced)
Fresh basil (chopped)	
Fresh cilantro (chopped)	Pine nuts
Fresh mint (chopped)	Pumpkin seeds
Fresh parsley (chopped)	Sesame seeds
	Sunflower seeds

Dressings (pick one)

Asian Ginger Vinaigrette (page 271)	Olive oil
Balsamic vinegar	Savory Garlic Dressing (page 272)
Oil and lemon juice	

cod liver oil, borage oil, evening primrose oil, or flax oil. While all oils begin to smoke at a different temperature, it is important to ensure that they never reach that point during cooking. Once an oil hits its smoke point, it is biochemically altered and is no longer healthy. Instead of helping to alleviate inflammation in your body, it will actually cause it.

Most grocery store oils have been heated and denatured extensively before even arriving at the store, making them rancid and unhealthy choices. They should be completely avoided.

Milk and Milk Substitutes

You'll learn below about the acid-forming properties of cow's milk. However, there are many delicious and easy-to-use alternatives. Goat's milk is alkalizing, as are coconut milk and almond milk. Goat's milk should still be consumed in moderation as it can be mucus forming and clog the body's lymphatic system, which is so important to weight loss (check out Tip #41 on page 175 for more information about the importance of the lymphatic system and how to ramp it up for weight loss).

Coconut milk contains medium-chain triglycerides—a type of natural, healthy fat that helps boost your thyroid gland's functioning. Your thyroid gland is the seat of much of your metabolism, making its ability to function well imperative to weight loss. Check out Tip #19 (page 129) for more information about coconut oil and Tip #42 (page 177) for more information about boosting your thyroid gland if it is underactive. Choose unsweetened coconut milk to use in tea, in smoothies, or as a substitute for milk in recipes. I'm referring to the cartons of coconut milk for drinking, not the thicker coconut cream found in cans, although preservative-free coconut cream is excellent on the 60 Seconds to Slim program and a delicious addition to curries, soups, or stews. Enjoy my recipe for Thai Ginger-Coconut Soup, found on page 261.

Unsweetened almond milk is high in calcium and magnesium, two important alkaline minerals that help to alkalize your body. Enjoy it on cooked quinoa for breakfast, in a smoothie, or in place of milk in recipes. You can purchase it or you can make your own. Check out my recipe for Alkalizing Almond Milk on page 246 if you wish to make it yourself.

Water, Water Everywhere

Drink lots of water to flush excess acidity and toxins from the body. That means alkaline water (most tap water and bottled water is acidic).

Q&A Timing Your Water Intake

Q. Why should I drink water 20 minutes before meals?

A: You'll be drinking a lot of water on this plan, which is imperative to flush fat and toxins from your body and to alkalize your body chemistry. However, it's best not to drink much water or other liquid with meals. Just drink enough to take any supplements or pills you need to take with food. Ideally, drink no later than 20 minutes before a meal and no earlier than 1 hour after a meal. Of course, these are just guidelines and you should never allow your body to become dehydrated. Make sure that you're drinking plenty of water when you wake up and between meals.

There are two big reasons for not drinking much with meals.

1. Drinking water between meals and up to 20 minutes before a meal keeps you fuller so you'll eat less food at mealtimes.

2. The liquid dilutes your stomach's hydrochloric acid and digestive enzymes needed in full strength for proper digestion. Drinking with meals only weakens digestion. Your stomach acid needs to remain at a low pH to adequately digest any protein foods you've eaten. When you drink liquids with meals, the pH is prematurely raised, falsely signaling your stomach to move its contents into the next phase of digestion in the small intestines. The small intestines cannot and should not do the work of the stomach. Over time, this mechanism can cause insufficient digestion. Whole food molecules can find their way into the intestines, where they can irritate the lining of the intestines, cause inflammation in the body if they find their way through the lining into the bloodstream, and cause nutrient deficiencies. That's because the intestines are the sites of nutrient absorption; however, if the food hasn't been broken down sufficiently to release its nutrients, a person will likely become deficient in critical nutrients, which can cause a whole array of symptoms depending on the specific deficiencies. Conversely, when food molecules enter the bloodstream, the immune system goes on alert, attacking them, which can result in serious illnesses if continued over time.

Alkaline water can be made cheaply by adding pH drops, powder, or fresh lemon to water. Lemon may seem acidic, but it has an alkalizing effect on your body.

Drink at least 1 quart (or liter, as they are close to the same measure) of water for every 50 pounds of your current body weight up to about 5 quarts or liters daily. (So, for a 150-pound person, that's 3 liters.) Add about 20 pH drops per cup of water (follow manufacturer's instructions). I'll further discuss pH drops momentarily. The water can be hot or cold but add the pH drops after heating if you're using hot water. Timing is also important. Ideally, wait at least 20 minutes before eating your next snack or meal and at least an hour after eating before having your next drink of alkalizing water. Drinking enough water is an essential part of the 60 Seconds to Slim Plan. You can't flush fat out of your body without sufficient water intake. I emphasize this element of the plan so heavily because I discovered that many people who followed the program just didn't get the message about water being so critical. I found them following the food suggestions and not drinking enough water—and not getting any results. Don't be like them: Keep a pitcher of water handy at all times, and you will achieve better results.

Condiments and Spices

Unlike table salt, which has been excessively refined and is acid forming, unrefined sea salt like Celtic sea salt is alkalizing. So is Himalayan crystal salt. Most fresh and dried herbs are alkalizing, including basil, ground red pepper, cilantro, oregano, parsley, rosemary, sage, and thyme.

Supplements on the 60 Seconds to Slim Plan

Choosing a lifestyle that supports a healthy and thin weight can be as simple as alkalizing your body. As you learned earlier, acid and alkaline are opposite sides of the biochemical spectrum. Supplementing your mostly alkaline diet with specific nutritional supplements can help restore the balance. While supplements are not a substitute for a healthy diet and lifestyle, they can assist you in making your body more alkaline. I recommend some specific ones as part of a healthy lifestyle, including green food powders and pH drops or powder. I suggest other specific weight-loss supplements later in the plan, but for now it is beneficial to use both of these supplements.

Most people expect to obtain all of their nutrients from food. And in an ideal world, that would be possible. But most of our food is depleted of essential vitamins and minerals because of overfarming, transportation, and other issues that affect its nutrient content. Additionally, few of us eat the ideal diet. That's why I recommend green food powder and alkalizing pH drops or powder. The first is a natural food supplement, and the latter is usually made up of essential minerals often missing or insufficient in the diet. While not mandatory, you'll most likely get better health and weight-loss results if you include them as often as you can. While you might find some good-quality options in your local pharmacy, your health food store is likely to have superior ones. And, as with your food, read labels. One of my clients wasn't getting good results, so she brought in her bag of supplements. They were full of artificial colors, sweeteners, flavors, and fillers. Avoid supplements that contain these harmful artificial substances.

GREEN FOOD POWDERS

There are many different kinds of green powders, primarily made from spirulina or chlorella algae and the juices of various grasses: barley, wheat, or alfalfa. These ingredients might seem like a recipe for swamp water, but add a teaspoon or two to water, juice diluted with water, or a smoothie and you'll be surprised how good they can taste. More important, they help alkalize your body, thereby promoting greater energy, pain resistance, and resistance to illness. If you don't like one type, choose a different kind, since there is a significant variation in taste between green powders.

PH DROPS AND POWDERS

Special formulations designed specifically for balancing your body chemistry are on the market. As with anything, there is a huge variation in the quality of these products, so it may take some experimentation to see which one works best for you. They usually contain a solution of chlorine dioxide or hydrogen peroxide, which releases oxygen in your body, helping to restore biochemical balance. Sometimes the powders contain a variety of alkaline mineral salts, namely potassium, magnesium, manganese, calcium, and iron. Follow package instructions for use. Note that pH drops are sometimes labeled as aerobic oxygen, oxygen, alkaline balance, or sodium chloride drops.

Eliminating Barriers to Fat Loss

Now that you know which foods speed weight loss and revitalize your health, we must also discuss foods you'll need to replace or cut drastically if you want to see results. In the last chapter, you assessed your diet and lifestyle and may have been shocked to see your results when testing your urine or saliva pH. Let's start exploring some of the main culprits that lead to acidity and excess weight so you can eliminate them from your diet. These are the foods that act as barriers to weight loss. It doesn't matter how many healthy choices you make or how much you work out—if you keep eating foods that are extremely acid forming in your body, you will throw off your blood sugar balance, increase the detoxification workload of your liver and kidneys, and cause your body to hoard fat. Foods either support your health or they destroy it and sabotage your efforts to achieve or maintain a healthy weight. The following foods are among the worst you can eat if you want to lose weight and have vibrant health. Of course, they need to be eliminated from your diet.

Top 10 Foods That Sabotage Your Weight-Loss Efforts

Let's face it: Grocery and convenience stores (not to mention school lunchrooms and vending machines) are full of chemical- and sugar-laced foods we should never eat but that make up a surprisingly large portion of most people's regular diet. I'm frequently asked which foods are the worst and make us the fattest. Here are 10 of the worst foods you may be eating, ordered from terrible to tragic. You may be surprised to learn which "food" I consider to be the worst.

10. **Ice cream.** I'm sure you're not surprised to see ice cream on this list, but it may not be for the reasons you think. Today's ice cream is full of sugar and harmful trans fats as well as artificial colors and flavors, many of which are proven neurotoxins that should never be allowed in food. Neurotoxins are brain- and nervous system–damaging chemicals. You may think that neurotoxins won't have an effect on your weight, but they certainly do. Our brains must maintain a delicate balance of chemicals that control all of our metabolic processes. If any substance

interferes, the balance goes out of whack. Of course, there are healthier varieties of ice cream, but most ice cream is hazardous to your health and weight. The best way to indulge without exposing yourself to dangerous chemicals is to make your own ice cream from scratch. It's not as hard as it sounds, and I've included a recipe for Strawberry Coconut Milk Ice Cream on page 295 for you to try.

9. **Corn and tortilla chips.** Since the advent of genetically modified foods, most of the corn we eat is a health-damaging Frankenfood. That's because corn is one of the most genetically modified foods grown. Because of its high sugar content, corn causes rapid blood sugar fluctuations, which translate into fat hoarding and weight gain, as well as mood swings, irritability, and many other symptoms. Most chips are fried in oils that have turned rancid and are linked to inflammation.

8. **Pizza.** While not all pizza is bad, most of the commercially available and frozen pizza on the market is full of artificial dough conditioners and preservatives. It is made from white flour that has been bleached and reacts in your body just like sugar, causing weight gain and blood sugar imbalances. Contrary to what dairy marketing boards will tell you, cheese is not a health food. Most cheese is high in saturated fats and is heavily processed.

7. **French fries.** Not only do french fries typically contain trans fats that have been linked to a long list of diseases, but they also contain one of the most potent carcinogenic substances in food—acrylamide. Acrylamide is formed when white potatoes are heated at high temperatures, such as during frying. Acrylamide can cause inflammation in your body and throw off its pH balance in favor of acidity. Additionally, most of the oils used for frying turn rancid in the presence of oxygen or at high temperatures—yet another way these foods can cause inflammation in the body. And researchers are discovering that inflammation is a factor in many serious health conditions, including heart disease, cancer, and arthritis, and, of course, weight gain.

6. **Potato chips.** You may not be surprised to see potato chips on this list, but it may surprise you to learn that, according to Health Canada, potato chips typically contain the highest levels of toxic acrylamide of any food. If you, like many people, crave potato chips, don't worry: I'll teach you what your cravings mean on page 74 and give you delicious and satisfying alternatives to these harmful snacks.

5. Bacon. Yes, bacon! Sorry, bacon lovers. According to research in the journal *Circulation*, daily consumption of processed meats like bacon can increase the risk of heart disease by 42 percent and diabetes by 19 percent. Bacon is full of nitrites, is loaded with salt, and is seriously acid forming. Contrary to what some diet plans teach, bacon has no place in a weight-loss program, or any health program for that matter. Not convinced? Before you say yes to bacon, consider the other health effects of eating it. A study at the University of Columbia found that eating bacon 14 times a month was linked to damaged lung function and a significantly increased risk of lung disease. Remember, no weight-loss program should cause weight loss at the cost of your overall health. Yet that is exactly what many high-protein diets do, particularly when they include regular bacon consumption as part of their meal plan.

4. Hot dogs. Questionable contents aside, even the 100 percent beef variety is bad for you. A study at the University of Hawaii found that consumption of hot dogs and other processed meats increased the risk of pancreatic cancer by 67 percent.[1] One of the ingredients found in both bacon and hot dogs is sodium nitrite. This carcinogen has been linked to leukemia in children and brain tumors in infants. Other studies show that sodium nitrate also promotes colorectal cancer.[2]

3. Doughnuts. Compared with prepackaged snack foods, a fresh doughnut may not seem bad, but most doughnuts are 35 to 40 percent trans fats—the worst kind of fat you can eat. Trans fats are linked to obesity and heart and brain diseases as well as cancer. And then there are the sugar and artificial dough conditioners and food additives many doughnuts contain. As if that weren't bad enough, the average doughnut also contains about 300 calories. If you're craving a sweet, try one of the dessert recipes in Part 3 and you'll never look back!

2. Soda. According to research reported by Dr. Joseph Mercola, "one can of soda has about 10 teaspoons of sugar, 150 calories, 30 to 55 milligrams of caffeine, and is loaded with artificial food colors and sulphites."[3] That alone should make you rethink your soda habit. But soda is also extremely acidic. It takes over 30 cups of pH-balanced water to neutralize the acidity of one cola. This acid residue can be extremely hard on the kidneys since they have to filter it. Additionally, the bones act as mineral reservoirs. Alkaline minerals, like calcium, are dumped into the blood to help neutralize acidity, which can weaken the bones over time. And, of course, the 10 teaspoons of sugar are a serious culprit in weight gain. In studies, soda is also linked to osteoporosis, obesity, tooth decay, and heart disease. If you're thinking of switching to diet soda, keep reading.

1. **Diet soda.** Diet soda is the winner of the Worst Food of All Time Award. Not only does diet soda have most of the problems of regular soda, but it also contains aspartame, now called AminoSweet. According to research by Lynne Melcombe, author of *Health Hazards of White Sugar*, aspartame is linked to the following health conditions: anxiety attacks, binge eating and sugar cravings, birth defects, blindness, brain tumors, chest pain, depression, dizziness, epilepsy, fatigue, headaches and migraines, hearing loss, heart palpitations, hyperactivity, insomnia, joint pain, learning disabilities, PMS, muscle cramps, reproductive problems, and even death.[4] Aspartame's effects can be mistaken for Alzheimer's disease, chronic fatigue syndrome, epilepsy, Epstein-Barr virus, Huntington's chorea, hypothyroidism, Lou Gehrig's disease, Lyme disease, Ménière's disease, multiple sclerosis, and post-polio syndrome. It still astounds me that some diet programs include this treacherous beverage as a means to lose weight. This is pure propaganda and lobbying on the part of the manufacturers and not based in fact. I know many people whose abilities to lose weight improved only after they cut out the diet soda. I also know people whose migraines and heart palpitations—and even a brain tumor—disappeared after they cut out diet soda. This is not food, and it has no place in your diet.

All of these foods are highly acid forming and need to be eliminated as soon as possible. They create inflammation in the body, throw off hormonal balance, bog down the body's lymphatic system (more on that later), and congest the liver, among other things that negate your efforts to restore a healthy weight.

Ditch the Three Ps: Processed, Prepared, Packaged

By eliminating the Top 10 Foods That Sabotage Your Weight-Loss Efforts, you'll take giant leaps toward improving your diet. The next step is to eliminate the Three Ps: processed, prepared, or packaged foods. Now, of course, a package of legumes or quinoa is not the same as the vast majority of packaged food you'll find in most grocery stores. The latter are bombarded with harmful ingredients that acidify your body, have addictive effects, and congest your detoxification organs. When it comes to the Three Ps, here's what you need to know.

Read Labels

Start reading labels. Some people look at this as a time waster, but it's important to view it as an opportunity to empower yourself with information. You'll be shocked to learn just how much junk is in your food, including trans or hydrogenated fats, sugar, high fructose corn syrup, artificial sweeteners, artificial flavors, flavor enhancers, texturizers, artificial colors, and many other harmful things that just don't belong in our food supply.

You may be surprised to learn that the average person eats 124 pounds of food additives every year.[5] Now that you understand that the vast majority of these synthetic ingredients are acid forming and, as a result, have an affinity for fat, you'll better understand why increasing studies are showing that we are storing these harmful toxins in fat deposits on our bodies. According to Dr. Patricia Fitzgerald, author of *The Detox Solution*, "Each year, the EPA [US Environmental Protection Agency] performs a study of the chemicals found in human fat tissue samples. DDT continues to be found in 100 percent of the tissue examined."[6] This is interesting because DDT was banned in the United States and Canada 30 years ago.

Begin by eliminating foods with ingredient names that you cannot pronounce or understand. That could include sodium benzoate, partially hydrogenated vegetable oil, or FD&C number 5. Let's face it: They don't sound appetizing anyway.

Reading labels will also help you moderate your intake of sugar, monosodium glutamate (MSG), saturated fats, sodium, and other foods that I discuss in greater detail over the next few pages.

Sift Out Sugar

Would it surprise you to know that the average person eats more than 2½ pounds of sugar each week? For some people, that is like eating their entire body weight in sugar every year. Most people eat as much sugar in 2 weeks—5 pounds—as our ancestors did in an entire year a century ago. We are a society of sugar addicts who don't recognize the harmful effects of eating so much of the sweet white stuff. It is one of the most dangerous substances to enter our body, especially when eaten in such high quantities.

While it's fairly obvious that sugar is found in soft drinks, sweetened juices, cookies, cakes, and pastries, it is also hidden in many other foods. And while it's one of the worst culprits for weight gain, that is not the only health issue it poses.

Sugar is linked to high blood pressure, heart disease, diabetes, premature aging, high cholesterol, and of course, weight gain. If you suffer from unusual mood swings, depression, allergies, or hormonal imbalances, look at your sugar consumption first. These symptoms may be linked to the cakes, cookies, ice cream, concentrated fruit juices, and other sweet treats that pervade our diet. But don't stop there. Sugar is an insidious toxin, hidden in surprising quantities in food items like ketchup, meat, french fries, and even salt. That's right. Many brands of salt contain sugar, probably because sugar is so addictive. Some experts indicate that it is more addictive than cigarettes. It's everywhere, and it is making you sick and overweight.

Soda is arguably the worst source of sugar in the modern diet. The average man, woman, and child in the United States drinks about 848 cups of soda every year—that's 600 servings of liquid sugar—in the form of cola, root beer, and lemon-lime and orange-flavored soda, to name a few. Each beverage alone contains 7 to 11 teaspoons of sugar. While adults should know better, soda has become the beverage of choice for the last couple of generations of children, and it is wreaking havoc on their bodies. Not only does sugar contribute to the health problems mentioned above (and others), but soda is also highly acidic, which further compromises the body's ability to function properly. The average can of Coca-Cola measures 2.52 on the pH scale, where 0 is the most acidic and 14.0 is the most alkaline. You can see that Coke is pretty acidic!

And don't think Pepsi or other types of soda are superior. According to research by Dr. Robert O. Young, Pepsi measures 2.61 on the pH scale, only modestly better than Coke and not enough to be a good choice for your health or weight. Orange soda is 2.9, Mountain Dew is 3.27, Sprite is 3.29, and root beer is 4.24.[7] No matter what type of soda you drink, and this includes carbonated water (sorry, seltzer fans), it is extremely acid forming, and it is damaging your body and contributing to your weight gain.

As I mentioned above, it takes more than 30 glasses of pure, neutral water (most tap water is acidic) just to neutralize the acidity in a single glass of regular or diet soda.[8] That's because, in addition to either acidic sugar or artificial sweeteners, the main ingredient in soda is phosphoric acid, which registers 2.8 on the pH scale—highly acidic. Research links phosphoric acid to osteoporosis because of its tendency to leach calcium and other minerals from the bones and to prevent minerals from being absorbed in the body. Now that you know that the bones are the reservoirs of calcium for neutralizing acidity, I'm sure you'll understand how phosphoric acid has this effect on the body.

Additionally, the body uses fat stores to keep acids, including phosphoric acid, out of the blood circulation. So you can see how soda quickly contributes to excess weight and poor health. While it may be a good thing to keep acids out of your bloodstream, it's not really a consolation if you're packing on extra pounds.

While clean, pure alkaline water is the ultimate beverage for the human body, you can enjoy many other delicious beverages, including herbal teas and other power-packed drinks that will increase your energy and help you drop pounds. I include a few recipes in this book that will help quench your thirst. Instead of cola, coffee, or black tea, try my recipe for Super Fat-Busting Green Tea Lemonade on page 245. It's delicious, a cinch to make, and helps burn fat, unlike the other options.

If you're reading labels, you'll find sugars hiding under names that end in -ose, particularly high fructose corn syrup. There are many others, including dextrose, maltose, lactose, and fructose. Many are touted as "natural sweeteners." While they may be preferable to artificial sweeteners, they still cause your body to gain weight. If you want to lose weight, lose the sweeteners.

The positive news is that it's fairly easy to reduce sugar consumption because we eat so much of it. So, this week, eliminate soft drinks, cakes, pastries, fruit juices, and other sugary foods. Don't worry—you'll be replacing these harmful foods with truly delicious and satisfying foods that will make you forget you ever craved these health destroyers. When one of my clients tried Super Fat-Busting Green Tea Lemonade, she couldn't believe how easy it was to give up her cola habit. And the recipe for Strawberry Coconut Milk Ice Cream (see page 295) is so good you'll never look back at the artificial version. Change can sometimes feel difficult, but I am hoping you will see it for what it truly is—a giant leap to improve your life. I love the quotation from Thomas Edison, "Opportunity is missed by most people because it is dressed in overalls and looks like work." I will be asking you to eat differently and to do a bit more exercise than you may have been doing up to this point. I hope you will see the effort for what it truly is: an opportunity to transform your life. Later in this chapter I'll explain how to

Exposed Sugar Sources

You may be shocked to discover sugar's hiding places. Here are a few surprising sources:

- Sugar is added to lunchmeats, canned meat, and bacon to add flavor and keep them looking pink longer than they normally would.
- Some brands of salt contain sugar.
- Most commercial condiments such as ketchup and mustard are largely sugar.
- Just prior to slaughter, many animals are fed sugar to "improve" the flavor and color of their meat.
- Poultry is frequently injected with sugar solutions to add flavor—especially at many fast-food restaurants.
- Most commercial brands of peanut butter are loaded with sugar.
- Alcoholic beverages, including wine, beer, mixed drinks, and champagne, are high in sugar.
- The breaded coating on most foods contains sugar.
- Corn syrup or molasses is often added to the hamburger served in many restaurants to reduce shrinkage during cooking.
- Most canned salmon receives a sugar glaze prior to canning.
- Bouillon cubes for making soup usually contain sugar.
- Dry cereals are notorious sources of large amounts of sugar.
- The canned cranberry sauce and cranberry "juice" sold at most grocery stores are about 90 percent sugar.

decode your cravings and, more important, how to eliminate them. For now, be sure to read "Exposed: Sugar Sources," below, to discover many unexpected ways sugar creeps into your diet. If you're disheartened by this list, be sure to check out all the mouthwatering foods you can eat in the recipe section.

BLOOD SUGAR BALANCING

When it comes to sugar, eating less of it is not the only important factor in weight loss. Balancing your blood sugar levels is also one of the most critical factors in whether you will lose weight or not. Whole books have been written on the topic, but fortunately it's not necessary to read one to balance your blood sugar. I'll simplify the topic for you here.

When you eat sugar or something sweet or even refined starchy foods and white potatoes, your blood sugar levels skyrocket. To cope, your pancreas secretes the chemical insulin to help deal with the sugar and to prevent the high level of glucose from damaging your brain or other organs. The insulin helps to reduce the blood sugar levels, but it also effectively tells your body to hoard fat. Your blood sugar drops, you crave something sweet or high in carbohydrates, and the insulin response is triggered all over again. If this cycle continues, your body may stop responding properly to insulin, which creates a condition known as insulin resistance. If not attended to through diet and exercise, insulin resistance can lead to metabolic syndrome. I'll discuss this condition more in depth momentarily. But first let's look at a condition called "hypoglycemia."

I'm always astounded how many clients come in and tell me that they are "hypoglycemic" and that their doctors have told them to eat white sugar when they feel hypoglycemic. Their doctors have obviously taken a blood test—a snapshot of a particular moment in time—and given them this ominous-sounding diagnosis. The clients come into my office in a panic, sometimes almost proud that they know this medical jargon. But this diagnosis is not the whole story.

Hypoglycemia comes from the Greek *hypo* (meaning "low" or "under") and *glycemia* ("blood sugar"). Everyone has low blood sugar at various times because we skip meals, eat refined sugar, eat excessive amounts of sweets and refined carbohydrates, and don't eat often enough.

Whether you are aware of having low blood sugar, want to lose weight, or sometimes crave sweets, balancing blood sugar levels is essential.

How to Balance Your Blood Sugar Levels for Weight Loss

1. Stop eating refined sugars and foods made with them. That includes soda, juices, and starches like white bread, white pasta, white potatoes, and white rice.

2. When you eat carbohydrates, choose whole grains, seeds, nuts, and vegetables.

3. Eat some healthy protein, beneficial fats, and fiber at every meal.

4. Eat a meal or snack every 2 to 3 hours. Do not skip meals.

Danger: Metabolic Syndrome

Metabolic syndrome is increasingly common in overweight and obese individuals. Also called syndrome X, metabolic syndrome is a collection of symptoms linked with insulin resistance. While it can occur on its own, this is rare. More often insulin stops being effective in promoting the transport of sugar from the blood to the muscles or tissues, where it is needed for energy. Metabolic syndrome is linked to high blood pressure, cholesterol abnormalities, and increased risk of blood clotting. According to the World Health Organization, metabolic syndrome is determined by all of the following:

- High insulin levels after fasting or after meals
- Abdominal obesity, which is a waist measurement over 37 inches
- High triglyceride levels (at least 150 mg/dL) or HDL cholesterol levels lower than 35 mg/dL
- High blood pressure (140/90 mmHg or above), or being treated for high blood pressure

By following the 60 Seconds to Slim program, you'll be eating less refined sugar, exercising more often, balancing your pH and your blood sugar levels, and eating healthier food. In other words, you'll be making great strides toward reducing or eliminating your risk of experiencing metabolic syndrome.

If you fail to balance your blood sugar levels, you will not have the weight-loss results you'd like. It's that simple. Unless you have a serious health condition like diabetes, balancing your blood sugar will happen almost immediately if you follow the above recommendations. The rewards for stabilizing your blood sugar are many: more energy, fewer afternoon slumps, balanced moods, clearer thinking, and of course, weight loss.

WINNING SUGAR SUBSTITUTIONS

Instead of sugar or artificial sweeteners, *Stevia rebaudiana*, or stevia as it is usually called, is the best natural sweetener to choose. It is the only sweetener that doesn't impact blood sugar levels, the process that causes fat hoarding in your body. It is an herb that just happens to taste sweet, but not from sugar content. It actually tastes between 300 and 1,000 times sweeter than sugar, depending on the form you use—the whole herb, the powder, or the liquid extract. I recommend the whole herb, which is usually ground into a greenish powder, or the liquid extract. Most people prefer the liquid extract.

Stevia can be found in most health food stores and many traditional grocery stores as well. This is a natural product, and it will vary in taste from one manufacturer to another. I find that the liquid drops have less aftertaste than the powder or the whole herb. If you aren't crazy about the taste of one stevia product, don't give up. Try a different brand. Not all tomatoes or apples taste the same—the same holds true for stevia. I use about 1 or 2 drops of liquid stevia in my herbal tea, and it makes a sweet, warm treat.

If you just can't eliminate sugar and won't use stevia, palm sugar and coconut sugar (or coconut sap, as it is also called) are the next best choices to help you lose weight. They contain fewer grams of sugar per teaspoon and contain minerals to help support their digestion and absorption. My third choices include unpasteurized honey (purchased from a local beekeeper or natural food store only, since most grocery store brands don't actually contain honey but are simply sugar cocktails) or pure maple syrup. However, these natural sweeteners are still high in natural sugars and can contribute to weight gain, so use them sparingly. Whether you use palm or coconut sugar, honey, or maple syrup, use them in small amounts (no more than 1 teaspoon three times a day).

While these natural sweeteners are better than processed sugar and much better than artificial sweeteners, which I'll discuss momentarily, they will still cause blood sugar fluctuations and contribute to weight gain. If you can't make a clean break from these sweeteners, remember to use less than 1 teaspoon and don't use it more than three times a day. You won't lose as much weight if you keep these foods in your diet.

Whatever you do, do not replace sugar with artificial sweeteners, which is like replacing one poison with another.

A SWEETENER BY ANY OTHER NAME?

Maybe you think that the news above about sugar doesn't apply to you because you use artificial sweeteners, right? Wrong! If there is one thing worse than sugar, it's chemically derived, artificial replacements for sugar. The slick marketing campaigns, extensive lobbying, and catchy names have fooled many people, but the truth about these toxins cannot be covered up simply by changing the product name. If you think reaching for the diet cola is the lesser of two evils, think again. The list of health problems caused by these sugar substitutes is even longer than that of sugar.

Artificial sweeteners are known by their chemical names, such saccharin, aspartame, and sucralose. They are commonly used under their brand names: Neotame or AminoSweet, Sweet 'N Low, and Splenda. Read Tip #2 (page 91) and Tip #3 (page 95) to learn more about the artificial sugar substitutes and how they are contributing to your weight and health issues.

Make MSG M.I.A.

One of the most commonly used and most widely known food additives is monosodium glutamate (or MSG, as it is better known). MSG is a pervasive chemical that is added food to enhance its flavor. It is found in almost all restaurant food, not just Chinese food, and virtually all packaged, bottled, and prepared foods. Unfortunately, governments have not recognized the harmful and addictive nature of this substance, so it doesn't even need to be labeled as monosodium glutamate.

In fact, it has many guises, including:

Autolyzed yeast

Calcium caseinate

Gelatin

Glutamate

Glutamic acid

Hydrolyzed protein

Hydrolyzed soy protein

Monopotassium glutamate

Sodium caseinate

Yeast extract

Yeast food

Yeast nutrient

In addition to being linked with weight gain and an insatiable appetite, it is addictive. People don't feel full on MSG. Additionally, it is linked with many other health issues, including asthma, headaches, dizziness, nausea, diarrhea, a burning sensation of the skin, changes in heart rate, difficulty breathing, and anxiety.

By eliminating the Three Ps—processed, prepared, and packaged foods—as I suggested earlier, you eliminate the likely sources of MSG. But beware of bottled sauces, condiments, and spice mixes, as it often lurks there as well. It may seem hard to cut out these convenience foods, but you'll soon learn how easy it can be to make delicious, healthy food that supports your weight-loss goals.

MSG is highly acid forming and contributes to weight gain. Read Tip #10 (page 106) to learn more about the dangers and hidden sources of MSG so you can be sure to eliminate it from your diet.

Find Out Which Fats Make People Fat

Many people, even those in the health industry, have a tough time keeping good and bad fats straight. Generally, trans fats and hydrogenated fats are damaging. While some saturated fat may not be a problem, excessive amounts of saturated fats—those derived primarily from meat, poultry, and dairy products—are also unhealthy because they have no nutritional value and make our bodies more acidic.

Even natural oils that offer us health benefits can become unhealthy oils through processing, high temperatures, overexposure to oxygen, and hydrogenation. Heating oils during the processing phase or when we cook (as in frying and deep-frying) can break down the beneficial fatty acids and form compounds such as hydrocarbons, ketones, and aldehydes that increase acidity in our bodies. Various cooking oils have different "smoke points"—the temperature at which oil begins to smoke and lose its health benefits. Olive oil, for example, smokes at just under 325°F. Flaxseed oil's smoke point is so low that it should never be heated. The higher the smoke point, the hotter the oil can get without not only losing its health benefits, but also producing those body-damaging chemicals.

Still, I encourage you to limit the amount of food you eat that requires heated oils. Many of these products were heated in the processing phase and are already rancid by the time you purchase them. Processing oils often includes adding hydrogen atoms to healthy fat to saturate the fat molecule, turning unsaturated oil into saturated oil. This creates "hydrogenated" or "trans" fats, foreign invaders that our bodies were never intended to ingest or digest. These fats are an industrial creation and our ancestors a few generations back were never exposed to these harmful, acid-forming poisons.

Trans fats strain the liver, an important organ in detoxification. Our intestines have no way to break down or absorb these manufactured fats. In an effort to neutralize these products, the body wastes its alkalizing resources, such as calcium, potassium, and sodium. Trans fats must be avoided completely, so be cautious of most packaged, processed, and prepared foods. These are common hiding places for trans fats. Read Tip #4 on page 97 to learn more about trans fats and why you need to eliminate them from your diet.

Replace trans fats, margarine, butter, and vegetable oils and foods made with them with extra virgin olive oil and coconut oil. Both can be used in breads and baking and in cooking.

DON'T PASS THE MARGARINE . . . PASS ON THE MARGARINE

Here is another great marketing campaign at the expense of our health. For decades, margarine has been billed as a healthy alternative to butter. In fact, it is estimated that four times as many Americans use margarine than butter. Margarine is not healthier than butter—they must both be avoided in not only a weight-loss program but also a healthy eating regimen. Margarine is simply cheaper than butter—which explains its common use. However, it usually contains harmful trans fats like those you just learned about. In *60 Seconds to Slim*, I recommend using healthy alternatives to butter and margarine, such as olive oil, coconut oil, and flaxseed oil (the latter is not for cooking). Check out the recipe for Alkalizing Butter Substitute on page 249.

Select the Right Salt

There is a lot of controversy over whether salt is good for us or not. But the arguments should not be quite so simplistic. The *quality* of the salt plays a significant role in its health-promoting or health-destroying characteristics. Ordinary table salt or iodized salt has been highly refined until it becomes the stuff we find in most grocery stores, restaurants, and homes. During the refining process, the electrical potential of the salt is denatured to the point that it has little value to us.

Unrefined sea salt or unrefined crystal salt are good options, although I'd choose the former because crystal salt often contains lead along with all the beneficial minerals. Unrefined crystal salt is not the same as iodized kosher salt. Iodized salt has been heavily refined and is no longer a healthy food. Unrefined sea salt usually has a slightly grayish color due to the minerals present. The minerals in the salt balance our body's natural electrolyte stores.

Decoded Your Cravings

What do you crave? The saltiness of potato chips, the cool creaminess of ice cream, or the rich flavor of chocolate? Whatever you're longing for, it may be your body's way of letting you know you're missing valuable nutrients. Here's how to decode your cravings.

All Cravings. Most cravings are actually signals from our bodies that we are dehydrated, but we misinterpret them as hunger pangs. By drinking a tall glass of water first, you may be giving your body exactly what it wants and alleviate the craving altogether. By some estimates, 80 percent of people are chronically dehydrated. So before you reach for food to nix your cravings, quench them with some water. Then wait half an hour. More often than not, they'll be gone.

Sweets. If you crave sweets of almost any kind, you may be experiencing blood sugar fluctuations. Giving in to pie, candy, cake, or other goodies only makes the problem worse by causing blood sugar roller coasters that lead to more cravings. Instead, choose a piece of fruit—preferably one that's not loaded with natural sugars—when you're craving sweets. And, in general, choose more high-fiber foods like beans and legumes and complex carbohydrates like whole grains that keep your blood sugar stable.

Chocolate. Cravings for chocolate often indicate that your body may be deficient in magnesium. Many nutritionists estimate that more than 80 percent of the population is lacking in dietary magnesium, which may explain why so many of us reach for chocolate. While chocolate can contain beneficial antioxidants, they usually come alongside plentiful amounts of sugar. If you eat chocolate, be sure to reach for dark chocolate—about

Additionally, the sodium found in unrefined sea salt has the electrical potential intact, which helps to bathe our cells in beneficial sodium needed for life. It even helps to alkalize our bodies. Don't go crazy with salt but feel free to use unrefined sea salt in moderation throughout the 60 Seconds to Slim Plan.

STAY LEAN WITH THE RIGHT KIND OF PROTEIN

Contrary to what some popular diet programs may tell you, our ancestors ate only about 5 percent of their caloric intake as animal protein. That's much

---

75 percent cacao or higher—which is usually lower in sugar and higher in antioxidants. Additionally, eat foods high in magnesium, such as nuts, seeds, fish, and leafy greens.

Salty Foods. Cravings for salty foods like potato chips or popcorn often mean chronic stress may be taking a toll on your adrenal glands—the two triangular glands that sit atop the kidneys and give us energy and help us to cope with stress of all kinds. Getting on top of the stress in your life is essential. Try meditation, breathing exercises, or other stress management techniques. Research at the University of Utah in Salt Lake City showed that people who take a break to breathe deeply or meditate before reaching for salty snacks reduced their stress hormones by 25 percent and cut the bingeing in half.

Red Meat. Not surprisingly, cravings for red meat usually indicate an iron deficiency. Often people crave burgers or steaks. Menstruating women are especially vulnerable to iron deficiencies. Beans and legumes, unsulphured prunes, figs, and other dried fruits are high in iron. However, eat dried fruits in moderation, since they are high in sugar and are acid-forming foods. Too many of these foods will counteract your best weight-loss efforts.

Cheese. Cravings for cheese or pizza often indicate a fatty acid deficiency, which is common since few people get enough omega-3 fatty acids. Reach for raw walnuts, wild salmon, and flaxseed oil, and add ground flaxseeds to your diet.

less than the 40 percent of daily calories most people eat now (or 248 pounds of meat per person every year in the United States). Most nutrition experts will tell you that amount is much higher than needed, yet somehow people still believe they are at risk for developing a protein deficiency. They're far more likely at risk of an acid excess due to all this meat. Meat leaves an acidic residue in our bodies after it is metabolized. This is acid that our bodies must neutralize and eliminate. Does that mean you have to go vegetarian on *60 Seconds to Slim*? Of course not, unless you want to. The program is designed to be flexible. But there's no room for negotiation when it comes to eating too much animal protein. Getting 40 percent of your daily calories from meat, like people do on the Standard American Diet, is simply not healthy. Eating that much meat not only leaves a highly acidic residue in the body but also puts a strain on your digestive enzymes and the organs responsible for making them (your pancreas, liver, intestines, and stomach). Additionally, the high-protein diet proponents won't tell you that excessive protein gets converted into fat in the body the same way excessive carbs do. So eating lots of animal protein may not help your weight-loss efforts.

Diets high in meat are usually higher in the minerals iron, sulfur, and phosphorus, which leave an acidic ash in our tissues and blood. While these minerals are important for maintaining good health, our bodies must work hard to eliminate the acidic waste. We draw upon alkaline substances in our bodies like calcium and magnesium to do so.

If you choose to eat animal-based protein on the 60 Seconds to Slim Plan, I encourage you to choose fish. Ideally, eat fish at least three times a week. Always choose wild over farmed fish when available, since it tends to be lower in toxic residues such as mercury. Fish is high in natural fats that help break down fat stores in our bodies. While it is acidic, it is definitely a Wise Acid choice that can comprise up to 30 percent of your diet. The remaining 70 percent should be alkaline foods from the alkaline side of the food chart on page 42. If you choose to follow the 60 Seconds to Slim program as a vegetarian or vegan, or if you simply won't eat fish, be sure to supplement your diet with at least 1 to 2 tablespoons of flaxseed or hempseed oil daily. If you eat canned fish, be sure to choose a natural food store brand that is not sugar glazed, since this is a common practice in fish canning.

Next to fish, organic or hormone- and antibiotic-free poultry and eggs are the best options for animal protein. That includes chicken, turkey, and various types of eggs. The hormones found in traditional poultry and eggs disrupt your body's natural hormone balance in favor of weight gain, not weight loss. The antibiotics found in most of these foods also disrupt your bowel flora balance, which is essential for weight loss (see Tip #59 on page 215 for more information). If you're eating fish, meat, poultry, or eggs, be sure it is no more than 6 ounces or one egg per meal. The remaining foods should be vegetables. Make sure that at least 70 percent of every meal consists of vegetables. I'm not referring to calories or weight here. I'm talking about simply eyeballing your plate. Does it look like 70 percent of the food on it is alkaline vegetables?

Regardless of whether you choose to eat animal products or go vegan on 60 Seconds to Slim, make sure you eat protein foods at every meal and as part of every snack. You can also choose from a wide variety of vegetarian sources of protein:

- Avocado
- Coconut
- Legumes, such as kidney beans, black beans, navy beans, pinto beans, Romano beans, chickpeas, soybeans, edamame (green soybeans)
- Nuts (raw, unsalted), including almonds, Brazil nuts, cashews, macadamia nuts, pecans, pistachios, and walnuts
- Quinoa (see Tip #34 on page 158 for more information about this valuable superfood)
- Seeds, such as chia seeds, flaxseeds, hemp seeds, pumpkin seeds, sunflower seeds, and sesame seeds
- Soy products such as tofu, miso, and tempeh
- Dairy alternatives including almond milk, coconut milk, hemp seed milk, and soy milk

GOT MILK? DITCH THE DAIRY PRODUCTS

Most people, including many nutritionists, have been duped by powerful dairy lobbyist organizations into thinking that dairy products are health foods. After all, they contain high amounts of calcium, right? Well, they contain calcium, typically along with blood and pus. But that's not the only problem with milk and dairy products; when your body metabolizes them, they are acid forming. Our bodies are constantly striving for biochemical balance to keep our blood at 7.365 pH. Eating excessive acid-forming dairy products can actually work in reverse, causing our bodies to deplete calcium rather than absorb it for building strong bones. As you learned earlier, alkaline calcium is stored in the bones and released to combat excessive acidity in the body, including the acidity caused from eating dairy products. That explains why research continues to show that the countries whose citizens consume the most dairy products have the highest incidence of osteoporosis. That's good enough reason to avoid them, but there are plenty more.

We're the only species (other than those we domesticate) that drinks milk after infancy. And we're definitely the only ones drinking the milk of a different species. Cow's milk is intended for baby cows, which have the four stomachs required to digest it.

Today's dairy products are loaded with hormones that disrupt our natural hormonal balance and can cause weight gain. Not only are the hormones naturally present in cow's milk stronger than human hormones, but the animals are routinely given steroids and other hormones to plump them up and increase milk production. These hormones can negatively impact humans' delicate hormonal balance and cause us to pack on the pounds.

Most cows are fed substances that should never find their way into our bodies. Commercial feed for cows contains all sorts of ingredients, including genetically modified (GM) corn, GM soy, animal products, chicken manure, cottonseed, pesticides, and antibiotics—none of which is beneficial to our bodies, to say the least.

Dairy products clog our lymphatic and other bodily systems because of their mucus-forming nature. This means that when we eat them, our organs and organ systems will not necessarily be functioning at optimum levels, which is what we're trying to achieve throughout the 60 Seconds to Slim Plan. Dairy can also contribute to respiratory disorders, further reducing our ability to inhale the oxygen-rich air that alkalizes our blood.

If that's not enough reason to ditch the dairy, consider the research linking dairy products with the formation of arthritis. In one study on rabbits, Richard Panush, MD, professor of medicine at the Keck School of Medicine of the University of Southern California, was able to produce inflamed joints in the animals by switching their water to milk.[9] In another study, scientists observed more than a 50 percent reduction in the pain and swelling of arthritis when participants eliminated milk and dairy products from their diet.[10]

REDUCE COFFEE AND TEA

Both coffee and black, green, and white tea are acid forming, contrary to what some nutrition books state. Some claim that coffee is alkaline once it is metabolized by the body. That is simply a myth. It starts out acidic and has the same effect on your body. Reduce your coffee and tea intake to no more than one beverage a day. The exception here is green or white tea (read and follow Tip #17 on page 126). Green tea is an excellent weight-loss beverage, but count it as a Wise Acid food, which altogether should make up no more than 30 percent of your total diet. Add pH drops (learn more on page 59) to the tea after it's been brewed. Add fresh lemon juice if you like. If you prefer a sweeter drink, add a drop or two of liquid stevia.

Ideally, if you're going to be drinking any coffee or tea, do so within an hour of working out for the best weight-loss benefits. Regardless, you'll need to balance it out with a lot of alkaline water.

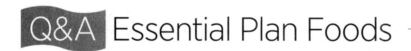

Q&A Essential Plan Foods

Q: What can I eat on this plan?

A: Don't be alarmed by the number of foods you'll be phasing out of your diet. Once you get going with the plan, you'll discover that there are many other foods you can eat, ranging from delicious nut, cheese, and bean spreads to decadent desserts and lots of things in between. You'll find that you can still eat many of your favorite foods, but you'll simply be learning new ways to make them. You'll find new favorites using ingredients with which you may not be familiar and explore delicious new recipes too. After you get used to this way of eating, you'll probably find that you prefer it. It just takes time to learn new food preparation techniques and to become familiar with new foods. For a better idea of what you'll be eating, make sure you check out the recipes starting on page 237.

The Importance of Exercise

Exercise is an integral part of the 60 Seconds to Slim Essential Plan. While you are following this plan, you'll be shaking loose a lot of acidic toxins that your body will need help flushing. Being active will help keep your bowels and your lymphatic system moving properly. Yes, exercise helps keep your bowels moving! If you are not already active, getting into a fitness routine is imperative to success on this plan.

In fact, developing a routine is important no matter how fit or active you currently are. If you are not very physically active, the transition doesn't have to be difficult: You can find time for an activity such as brisk walking at any time of day, at home, while traveling, or even at the office. As for strength training, lifting heavy books or grocery bags of food can work in the absence of weights or equipment, making this another portable and flexible way to boost your metabolism and burn more fat.

As the saying goes, "It's a poor carpenter who blames his tools." I believe that a lack of tools like exercise equipment is also a poor excuse for not exercising, especially when you pick activities that can be done anywhere.

Cardiovascular exercise

I want you to start doing some form of brisk walking, jogging, or other cardiovascular exercise for 30 minutes a day, at least 4 days a week. If you have been completely sedentary up until now, feel free to start with bouts of 10 minutes, adding 5 to 10 minutes each week until you are able to do 30. This is the minimum recommended amount of exercise needed to avoid gaining weight from being inactive—and a great place to start if your ultimate goal is to lose weight.

Strength training

On 2 days a week, also start weight training. This doesn't have to involve equipment if you don't have any. It could involve moves that force you to support your own body weight (such as pushups, leg lifts, and planks) or arm curls with bags of groceries or some other heavy item. Even 10 to 20 minutes of weight training twice per week will get you results. If you wish to do more, take at least 1 day off between training sessions to allow your muscles to recover. Try these basic strength-training moves:

- **Biceps Curls:** Grab a pair of weights and stand tall with your feet shoulder-width apart. Let the weights hang at your sides. Turn your arms so that your palms face forward. Without moving your upper arms, bend your elbows and curl the weights as close to your shoulders as you can. Pause, then slowly lower the weights back to the starting position. Each time you return to the starting position, completely straighten your arms. Complete 3 sets of 10 to 15 reps.

- **Overhead Triceps Extensions:** Grab a pair of weights and stand tall with your feet shoulder-width apart. Hold the weights at arm's length above your head, your palms facing each other. Without moving your upper arms, lower the weights behind your head until your forearms are parallel to the floor. Pause, then straighten your arms to return the dumbbells to the starting position. Complete 3 sets of 10 to 15 reps.

- **Chest Presses:** Grab a pair of weights and lie faceup on the floor with your knees bent and your feet flat on the floor. Hold the dumbbells above your chest with your arms straight. Lower the weights until your upper arms touch the floor, forming a 45-degree angle with the sides of your torso. Pause, then press the weights back up to the starting position. Complete 3 sets of 10 to 15 reps.

- **Body-Weight Squats:** Stand as tall as you can with your feet spread shoulder-width apart. Brace your core muscles, but note that your lower back should be naturally arched. Hold your arms straight out in front of your body at shoulder level. Lower your body as far as you can by pushing your hips back and bending your knees. Pause, then slowly push yourself back to the starting position. Keep your weight on your heels, not on your toes, for the entire movement. Complete 3 sets of 10 to 15 reps.

- **Knee Lifts:** Stand tall with your feet shoulder-width apart. Extend your arms straight out from your shoulders so that your body is forming a T shape. Lift your right leg up until your thigh is parallel to the floor and your leg is bent at a 90-degree angle. Slowly bring your right foot back down. Then lift your left leg in the same manner, as though you are marching in place in slow motion. Complete 3 sets of 10 to 15 reps.

- **Leg Lifts:** Lie flat on your back with your legs stretched out in front of you. If you feel uncomfortable or have back problems, try folding a towel and putting it under the curve of your back, just above your hips. Keeping your legs straight, slowly raise them until your body forms an L shape, with your toes pointed toward the ceiling. Slowly lower your legs to about an inch off the floor and pause before lifting them again. To make this move easier, try lifting one leg at a time, doing all reps on one leg before moving to the other. Complete 3 sets of 10 to 15 reps.

- **Horizontal Leg Lifts:** Lie on your left side, with your left elbow bent, cradling your head in your hand, and keeping your legs straight. Brace yourself with your right hand, palm down on the floor or mat. Raise your right leg as high as you can (this should take approximately 1 second) without moving any other part of your body, leaving your left leg firmly placed on the floor. Pause, then lower your leg back down (this should take approximately 3 seconds), and return to starting position. Complete 3 sets of 10 to 15 reps on each side.

As a general rule, be conscious of your posture when doing these moves and be careful not to strain your muscles. Respect your body and its limitations, particularly if you have any health issues. While it is important to go beyond your current boundaries, particularly if you are inactive, that doesn't mean harming yourself. As a rule of thumb, if a muscle feels sore, it's probably from lack of use; if a joint is sore, it may need some rest. And if it's swollen, ice may help.

Spend the next couple of weeks adjusting your fitness routine as needed to ensure that you are exercising for at least 30 minutes each day and doing strength moves twice a week. You will learn additional tips to ramp up your exercise and boost your fat-burning results in Week 3.

Q&A The 4-Week Plan

Now that you understand the basic tenants of the Essential Plan, it's time to read up on the 4-week plan. Here are a few quick questions and answers about this part of the program.

Q: Why are the tips grouped by week? Can I choose to do later tips earlier in the plan?

A: The tips are grouped into weeks because it's easier to make small changes gradually than to make lots of changes at once. If you overdo everything in Week 1, you'll likely feel overwhelmed and give up by Week 2. I have grouped tips into weeks by categories that are designed to help you focus on a particular area each week (for example, taking on new timing tricks one week while adding new supplements the following week). Each week builds on the achievements of the previous week. The first week focuses on foods to eliminate, because you won't see results if you don't cut your intake of those foods, which are acid forming and prevent your body from functioning at its best. However, when it comes to adding foods, supplements, and strategies, you can do 2 weeks at a time—or do all 65 tips at once, if you prefer. Just make sure you follow the minimum recommended at the beginning of each chapter. So follow all the suggestions outlined in the first week, at least five from Weeks 2 and 3, and two from Week 4.

Q: Why is there duplication between the tips? I've seen the same recommendation more than once.

A: You may notice some overlap in the foods, strategies, or supplements recommended. This is intentional and has been done for a number of reasons, including:

1. Certain foods are incredible for weight loss and need to be highlighted on their own because of their merits.
2. Many of those foods also belong on lists of top foods to increase weight loss, so you are likely to see them discussed at least twice, though you don't need to follow both tips.

(continued)

3. Certain foods are more like medicine for the glands and organs involved in weight loss, so any discussion of these glands or organs would be remiss without a discussion about critical foods to improve their function.

4. You will only be choosing a handful of tips each week, and I repeat certain items so you'll be more likely to choose them—and therefore improve your weight-loss results.

5. While I'd like you to follow the program as closely as possible, the repetition of specific foods presents another opportunity to include a food you may not have added to your diet yet.

Q: Why do we wait until Week 4 to add supplements if they have such dramatic results?

A: Supplements cannot stand in for a healthy diet. They are added in Week 4 to make the overall plan easier to follow; however, if you'd like to add them immediately or earlier in the program, by all means feel free to do that. The plan is structured to make it as easy as possible to switch from the Standard American Diet and fairly inactive lifestyle to a much healthier one. You may already be further along the spectrum, and it may be easy for you to jump in and add the supplements immediately. Do whatever feels right for you. However, if you need to make more dramatic changes to follow The Essential Plan and Week 1, I strongly recommend you wait on the supplements until you have developed the other healthy habits of this program.

Q: What do I do after the 4 weeks are over?

A: If you are ready to maintain your weight loss after 4 weeks, then you can stop doing the tips from the plan and just follow The Essential Plan to keep the weight off. If you have more weight to lose, you can continue on the 60 Seconds to Slim Plan, adding more tips as you go,until you reach your weight-loss goals. You can also continue on this program, with a bit more leniency if you prefer, for as long as you want to. Many people feel so good on the program that they choose to eat this way for life. Of course, you don't have to continue if you don't want to, but the health benefits of eating this way and following this lifestyle are many.

60 SECONDS TO SLIM
WEIGHT-LOSS TIPS

Part 2 contains the simple 60 Second substitutions, boosters, strategies, and supplements that supercharge your weight loss for optimum results. Add them to the Essential Plan over the next 4 weeks (or a shorter or longer period of time if you prefer).

Chapter 3

Week 1: SUBSTITUTE

The Foods to Avoid and the Foods That Will Replace Them

This week I will introduce you to the harmful foods and ingredients that may be causing you to gain weight. Many of these substances are hidden in common, everyday places. You learned about many of them in the previous chapter, but here you'll learn how to spot them, why you need to avoid them, how minimizing their consumption minimizes your waistline, and how to make simple substitutions so you don't feel deprived.

Here are the 60-Second Weight-Loss Tips you will learn in this section:

1. Ditch High Fructose Corn Syrup (page 89)

     Once you eliminate this sweetener from your diet, expect to see rapid weight loss.

2. Sayonara, Splenda (page 91)

     This artificial sweetener contributes to weight gain yet is hidden in most "sugar-free" products—and may even be hidden in your water supply.

3. Avoid Aspartame (page 95)

     Aspartame causes your body to pack on the pounds.

4. Take Out Trans Fats (page 97)

     Trans fats cause your body to hoard fat and fat deposits.

5. Say Goodbye to Soda—Even Diet Soda (page 98)

     Soda disrupts your body's natural biochemical balance and leads to weight gain.

6. Learn to Limit Sugar (page 100)

     Sugar quickly converts to fat in your body. Eating less of it goes a long way toward helping you achieve your desired weight.

7. Eliminate Suspected Food Sensitivities (page 102)

     Common food sensitivities can cause bloating and weight gain.

8. Don't Bother with Diet Pills (page 104)

     Diet pills contain the chemical phenylethylamine, which will make you binge once you stop taking them.

9. Don't Drink Diet Shakes (page 104)

     Glutamate, the protein in most weight-loss drinks, can actually make you fatter.

10. Uncover Hidden MSG (page 106)

     This common food additive causes you to feel hungry even when you're not.

11. Reduce Pesticides and Heavy Metals (page 109)

     Pesticides and heavy metals disrupt your body's natural fat-burning processes. Once you reduce your exposure, your body will be better able to rebalance.

12. Wipe Out White Flour (page 112)

     This particular type of carb leads to weight gain and dangerous blood sugar spikes.

60-Second Weight-Loss Tip #1:
Ditch High Fructose Corn Syrup

Once you eliminate this natural sweetener from your diet, expect to see rapid weight loss.

Corn syrup is the sugar extracted from corn. It is not and never has been healthy, but as corn is now almost entirely genetically modified, it is even worse for us. The fructose in high fructose corn syrup (HFCS) converts to fat stores quickly in your body, which is why it is frequently used in animal experiments to make animals obese. This food additive is found in most packaged, prepared, and fast foods and interferes with your body's appetite and metabolism hormones, causing your body to store fat. It can be found just about anywhere; food manufacturers have been profiting by sneaking this cheap food additive into our food supply in greater quantities over the last few decades, and it shows in our waistlines.

But there's good news. By eliminating the so-called natural sweetener for good, you can drop the weight and reduce high blood pressure linked to HFCS.

A University of Colorado study found that even people who eat a healthy, low-sodium diet may be at risk of high blood pressure because of this common food additive, which was shown to increase blood pressure by up to 32 percent.[1]

According to the study, HFCS leads to inflammation in the bloodstream, which causes the blood vessel walls to tighten, resulting in blood pressure increases. Even people who ate a healthy diet with periodic ingestion of HFCS experienced the blood pressure increase.

Another problem with the fact that HFCS is so commonplace in processed and prepared foods is that corn sensitivities are on the rise, affecting more people than ever. If you have developed a food sensitivity to corn, then continued exposure to it can cause bloating and weight gain—another great reason to give it up and slim your waistline.

HFCS can be listed on food labels as corn syrup, fructose, high fructose sweetener, natural sweetener, or even other types of sweetener, but it is still the same health-damaging ingredient. Even foods that claim to be "natural" can include HFCS. Only fresh whole foods are certain to be devoid of HFCS.

HFCS can be found in almost any foods but is common in most sodas and processed foods labeled "low fat" or "nonfat." (Most food manufacturers use high fructose corn syrup to add flavor when they make fat-reduced foods because it happens to be extremely cheap.)

Some surprising sources of HFCS include:

- Yogurt
- Baby food
- Granola and granola bars
- Cereal (even so-called healthy cereals or cereals intended for children)
- Salad dressing
- Condiments
- Crackers

As the name implies, high fructose corn syrup contains fructose, which is also found in fresh fruits. Research shows that consuming fruit does not negatively impact blood pressure, and may even improve it. However, if you see just the word *fructose* on a packaged food label, it most likely refers to HFCS and it will have the same harmful effect on your weight. Fructose found naturally in fruit can cause weight gain if eaten in high amounts, but fruit contains fiber and minerals like chromium that help slow sugar absorption. HFCS causes rapid blood sugar fluctuations and is a guaranteed way to gain weight.

How to Benefit

Read labels on any products you purchase and be sure that the ingredient list doesn't include high fructose corn syrup, corn syrup, or fructose. Though HFCS is present in many common foods, from loaves of bread to ketchup to fruit cups, chances are good that if the brand you usually pick includes HFCS, there's another brand on the same shelf or in your local health food store that doesn't. Don't just swap in foods containing sugar or artificial sweeteners, though, as you already know their harmful effects.

Super Health Bonus

There's another problem with HFCS: Most corn and corn-derived foods on the market are made with genetically modified (GM) corn. While there still isn't much testing on the effects of consuming GM foods (and certainly no long-term tests), early test results show many negative health consequences, including immune system disorders. So by eliminating HFCS, you'll reduce the likelihood of experiencing any potential ill effects of eating GM foods. Eliminating high fructose corn syrup will also help you to regulate blood pressure and triglycerides, two important factors for a healthy heart and arteries. By removing HFCS from your diet, you'll dramatically reduce your chances of suffering a heart attack or stroke.

60-Second Weight-Loss Tip #2:
Sayonara, Splenda

This artificial sweetener contributes to weight gain yet is hidden in most "sugar-free" products—and may even be hidden in your water supply.

A study conducted at Duke University and published in the *Journal of Toxicology and Environmental Health* found that sucralose (also known as Splenda):

- Is absorbed by fat cells (contrary to the manufacturer's claims about the artificial sweetener)

- Causes increases in body weight

- Reduces the amount of beneficial bacteria in your intestines by 50 percent (you'll discover later that this factor also contributes to weight gain, among other health issues)[2]

All of these effects of sucralose consumption can cause an increase in weight and fat and can sabotage your weight-loss efforts. Worse than that, sucralose is one of the main sweeteners used in "sugar-free" and "diet" foods and beverages. Many well-meaning dieters choose these options over foods with sugar to keep their weight down, but their efforts are being negated by this harmful artificial sweetener.

To make matters worse, new research shows that many people unsuspectingly drink sucralose every day in their water. A shocking new study found that the artificial sweetener is a widespread contaminant in surface water, groundwater, and wastewater. Researchers took samples from 19 American drinking water treatment plants that provide drinking water for over 28 million people. They found sucralose in:

- The source water of 15 out of 19 drinking water treatment plants tested
- The finished water of 13 out of 17 water plants
- Eight out of 12 water distribution systems[3]

Further, scientists determined that sucralose is a recalcitrant compound, meaning that it resists breakdown during chemical processes, including those involving chlorine at water treatment facilities.

The first question I'm typically asked when I tell my clients this information is, "Why is it allowed in our food and water?" That's a good question and one that is best directed to the Food and Drug Administration (FDA), Health Canada, and other similar regulatory bodies around the world. But let me tell you a bit more.

According to research by Dr. Joseph Mercola, the FDA conducted two human studies on sucralose prior to its approval of Splenda to determine whether it should be allowed in our food. The longest study lasted 4 days and examined only the effects of sucralose on tooth decay, not any other health effects. Additionally, when sucralose was tested to determine its absorption in the body, only eight men were studied. It is well known that this sample is too small to determine the health effects of any substance. It is also well known that women's and men's bodies may interact with a substance in a different way because of their significantly different hormonal systems. And, to state the obvious, 4 days is hardly enough time to determine safety! As for how it is allowed in our water—it isn't. Sucralose finds its way into our water supply because so many people are eating it and urinating it that it eventually finds its way into our drinking water.

What exactly is sucralose? Sucralose is not a calorie-free sugar that goes right through your body without being absorbed, even if that's what you've heard. It is not natural. It is a chlorinated artificial sweetener that was designed in a laboratory and is created in manufacturing facilities. Sucralose may start as a sugar molecule, but the similarities end there. Three chlorine molecules are added to each sugar molecule, which, according to Dr. Mercola, means that it "has been altered to the point that it's actually closer to DDT and Agent Orange than to sugar." So perhaps the manufacturer should start marketing it as the Agent Orange–Like Sugar That Can't Be Properly Metabolized by Your Body Because It More Closely Resembles a Horrendous Toxin—but that wouldn't sell much, would it?

Some of the symptoms linked with ingesting sucralose include:

- Allergic reactions such as facial swelling, swelling of the eyelids, tongue, throat, or lips
- Allergic skin reactions such as itching, swelling, redness, weeping, crusting, rashes, eruptions, or hives
- Anxiety
- Blood sugar increases
- Blurred vision
- Breathing problems including shortness of breath, coughing, chest tightness, and wheezing
- Depression
- Dizziness
- Gastrointestinal problems such as diarrhea, vomiting, nausea, bloating, gas, or pain
- Headaches
- Heart palpitations
- Itchy, swollen, watery, or bloodshot eyes
- Joint pains
- Mental fog
- Migraines
- Seizures
- Sinus congestion, runny nose, or sneezing
- Weight gain

How to Benefit

It is important to start reading labels on everything you purchase. (Of course, choosing fruits and vegetables in their unadulterated state means fewer labels to read, since produce usually doesn't require them.) Avoid any food that contains sucralose. Stop choosing diet beverages and adding packaged flavorings to your water. Avoid flavored water. Avoid "diet" or "sugar-free" baked goods, coffee syrups, and other items. That's the first step.

Getting sucralose out of the water you drink is a bit more difficult. If you have a reverse osmosis (RO) water filtration system, then you are filtering sucralose out of your water. This can be expensive and is not an option for everyone—however, giving up cable television for several months will pay for this type of water filtration system. And isn't your health worth more than sitting in front of the TV? Of course it is. If you're not prepared to purchase a reverse osmosis water filtration system, a carbon filter–based water filter will reduce the amount of sucralose you'll be exposed to. It is not as effective as an RO system but is much more affordable. The greater the amount of carbon the water passes through, the more effective the filter is at eliminating sucralose and other contaminants. And, of course, you must change your carbon filters regularly. Most of the pitcher-type systems require carbon filter changes every month.

So, if you can only afford a carbon filter–based water filtration pitcher, it's better than nothing. Drink filtered water instead of tap water every day. You can also save money by avoiding bottled water, which is no better than tap water. Actually, most bottled water is tap water from various city water supplies. And make sure the pitcher or bottles are bisphenol A (BPA) free. BPA is a harmful hormone disruptor found in many plastics.

Super Health Bonus

By eliminating sucralose from your diet, you'll likely experience other health benefits, including improved hormonal balance and fewer headaches or allergies.

60-Second Weight-Loss Tip #3:
Avoid Aspartame

Aspartame causes your body to pack on the pounds.

Shakespeare said, "A rose by any other name would smell as sweet." While that may be true of roses, it isn't true of artificial sweeteners. Aspartame recently had a name change in an effort to shake all the bad press linking it to a lengthy list of serious health conditions and is now known as Neotame and AminoSweet. These new names may sound sweet, but the chemical components of aspartic acid, phenylalanine, and methanol are just as harmful as ever. Humans have no enzymes in their bodies to break down methanol, so it gets converted into formaldehyde, a known carcinogen that most people have heard of but don't expect to ingest from their soda. This ultimately becomes formic acid, or formate, which significantly increases acidity levels in the body. You don't need to remember the biochemical chain of events that aspartame goes through once you've ingested it. You just need to remember that the by-products of trying to metabolize this toxin are harmful enough to cause cancer.

Let's consider the history of aspartame—er, I mean AminoSweet.

It was first developed in 1974, and by 1980 an FDA Board of Inquiry voted unanimously *against* approving aspartame for human consumption, but the vote was overruled by FDA commissioner Arthur Hull Hayes Jr. by 1983. Only a year after the approval, an FDA task force learned that some of the original data showcasing aspartame's safety had been falsified to hide results revealing that animals fed aspartame had developed seizures and brain tumors; however, the FDA maintained its approval of this product.

In 1983, the same year aspartame was approved for use in carbonated beverages, a neuroscientist reported in the *New England Journal of Medicine* that aspartame may increase body weight by stimulating a craving for calorie-laden carbohydrates.

By 1991, the National Institutes of Health had cataloged 167 adverse effects linked to aspartame use. In 1992, the US Air Force issued a warning to pilots not to fly after ingesting aspartame. And by 1994, the US Department of Health and Human Services had linked the artificial sweetener to 88 symptoms of toxicity.

Research confirms that aspartame is an excitotoxin—a substance that literally excites brain or nervous system cells until they die.

According to Lynne Melcombe, author of *Health Hazards of White Sugar*, research links aspartame to the following health conditions: anxiety attacks; appetite problems such as binge eating and sugar cravings; birth defects; blindness and vision problems such as blurred vision, bright flashes, and tunnel vision; brain tumors; chest pain; depression and emotional problems; dizziness and vertigo; edema; epilepsy and seizures; fatigue; headaches and migraines; hearing loss and tinnitus; heart palpitations and arrhythmia; hyperactivity; insomnia; joint pain; learning disabilities; memory loss; menstrual irregularities and PMS; muscle cramps; nausea; numbness of extremities; psychiatric disorders; reproductive problems; skin lesions; slurred speech; and uterine tumors. Research even links aspartame to death.[4] Aspartame's effects can be mistaken for Alzheimer's disease, chronic fatigue syndrome, epilepsy, Epstein-Barr virus, Huntington's chorea, hypothyroidism, Lou Gehrig's disease, Lyme disease, Ménière's disease, multiple sclerosis, and post-polio syndrome.

According to Randall Fitzgerald, author of *The Hundred-Year Lie*, some of the cancers linked to aspartame include brain, liver, lung, kidney, and lymphoreticular cancer.[5]

And here's a shocker: According to the authors of the book *Hard to Swallow*, when a diet drink containing aspartame is stored at 85°F for a week or longer, "There is no aspartame left in the soft drinks, just the components it breaks down into, like formaldehyde, formic acid, and diketopiperazine, a chemical which can cause brain tumors. All of these substances are known to be toxic to humans."[6] Some of these substances are directly linked to cancer.

Suffering from migraines? Think about the pain the next time you add AminoSweet to your coffee. Splenda, or sucralose, which is supposedly "made from real sugar," is not a good option either. (If you haven't already, read Tip #2 on page 91.) Sucralose has been chemically altered so your body doesn't recognize it as food—probably because it no longer resembles food in any way. Manufacturer-funded studies found it also was linked to migraines. While insufficient independent or long-term studies have been done to identify the full impacts of artificial sweeteners, the reality is that they just don't belong in your body. And remember: Artificial sweeteners are added to processed, packaged, prepared, and restaurant foods as well. Check labels carefully to ensure your diet is free of these toxins.

The chemical products above have no place in anyone's diet. Yet many people, including diabetics, are eating them. They don't contribute to weight loss. Worse, they are highly acid forming and upset the acid-alkaline balance that promotes health and healing. They can help you gain weight, but I'm sure you'd rather avoid that.

How to Benefit

Stop using any products labeled "sugar free" or "diet." In most cases these terms are used wherever aspartame is found. That includes diet soda, sugar-free coffee syrups, sugar-free cookies, diabetic treats, sugar-free pastries, and more. And when the product doesn't contain aspartame it usually contains sucralose, so either way, you benefit from removing these harmful artificial sweeteners from your diet.

Super Health Bonus

By eliminating aspartame from your diet, you'll likely reduce your risk of cancer and neurological disorders too. At the very least, you'll probably suffer fewer headaches.

60-Second Weight-Loss Tip #4:
Take Out Trans Fats

Trans fats cause your body to hoard fat and fat deposits.

By now you've probably heard of trans fats. Trans fats are fats that have been chemically altered during the manufacturing and processing of oils and are found in most processed, packaged, and prepared foods. These "plastic fats," as I call them, are almost impossible for your body to digest and for your liver to process, making them highly likely to be stored in your body.

Trans fats come primarily from partially hydrogenated oil or hydrogenated oils. In a recent study, researchers found that eating a daily diet that included 2.5 grams of trans fats in a single meal per day caused people to gain 30 percent more belly fat over 6 years than those people who avoided trans fats. That's about the amount of trans fats in most fast-food meals. Combined with monosodium glutamate (MSG), which I'll discuss in Tip #9 (page 104) and Tip #10 (page 106), you have a recipe for belly fat accumulation.[7] Yet trans fats and MSG frequently go hand in hand.

Fast-food meals aren't the only places trans fats hide. They are in many bakery goods, such as cookies, cakes, pies, and even so-called healthy breads. They are even found in some health food store goods, so be sure to start reading labels. Even when a product claims "zero trans fats" the government allows a small amount of these toxic fats to be hidden in your food.

How to Benefit

Read the Nutrition Facts on the packages of any food products you purchase. Choose only products that state "0 g trans fat." While you still may be exposed to small amounts, it's better than the higher quantities found in many products. Also, stop buying bakery goods that do not include this information. While they may not contain trans fats, more than likely they do. Also, read the ingredient list and look for "partially hydrogenated" or "hydrogenated" on the label. If a product contains either of these terms or "vegetable shortening," skip it. It contains fattening and health-harming trans fats.

Super Health Bonus

By eliminating trans fats, you're also reducing the likelihood of experiencing diabetes, since these harmful fats are linked to this serious condition.

60-Second Weight-Loss Tip #5:
Say Goodbye to Soda— Even Diet Soda

Soda disrupts your body's natural biochemical balance and leads to weight gain.

Soda is one of the worst culprits for weight gain. It also interferes with weight-loss efforts. If you're drinking soda, it's time to switch to a healthier option (I'll provide some suggestions in a moment). First, let's explore why soda is such a problem. There is no health value in soda. It has nothing positive to contribute to your body: It is full of synthetic colors, preservatives, sugar, artificial sweeteners, and other unhealthy ingredients.

It also contains excessive levels of phosphoric acid, the primary ingredient in cola and other sodas. The body uses calcium it leaches from the bones to convert phosphoric acid into a more stable form called phosphate. While many people think kidney stones are caused from excessive amounts of calcium, they are more likely due to a phosphate excess. If your body is pulling calcium from your bones to offset phosphoric acid, you can probably guess what will happen if this dangerous habit continues—bone demineralization and, potentially, osteoporosis.

As you learned in Chapter 1, you need to maintain a balanced pH for optimum health and to regulate weight. Kick the soda habit and you'll be well on your way to kicking excessive acid in your body. Cola rates between 2.52 and 2.61 on the pH scale. You may recall that 7.0 is neutral. Cola and other types of soda are extremely acidic. Plus, soda forms an overwhelming amount of acid once it is inside your body—acid that must be neutralized with valuable minerals and water. You need to drink 32 cups of water (and expend tremendous amounts of energy that would be better used elsewhere in your body) just to neutralize the acidity of *one* glass of soda. Skip the soda and not only will you have more energy, but you'll also stop sabotaging your weight-loss efforts.

You may be thinking, "But this doesn't apply to me since I drink diet soda." Diet soda is worse than regular soda. Not only is it extremely acidic, but it also contains aspartame, which is detrimental to your health (see Tip #3 on page 95).

How to Benefit

Stop drinking soft drinks. It takes time for your tastebuds to adjust, but they will adapt. If you absolutely must have something fizzy, mix a small amount of pure juice like pomegranate with some carbonated water. But you should try to eliminate all carbonated beverages from your diet over time. And if you haven't already gotten the message, definitely avoid diet soda and other aspartame-loaded foods and beverages. Aspartame is found in many diet products as well as a wide variety of prepared foods. Shockingly, it is also found in some multivitamins, supplements, and pharmaceutical drugs. Be aware that most products that state "sugar free" or "diet" on the label are actually just hiding places for aspartame.

If you are thirsty, drink water, herbal tea, or vegetable juice (check labels on the bottled brands—they can be full of sugar and salt too).

If you have a sweet tooth, reach for a piece of fruit. I find a delicious blend of green tea and lemonade made with brewed green tea, freshly squeezed lemon, and ice and sweetened only with stevia, to be a great thirst quencher.

Super Health Bonus

By forgoing soda, you're taking a huge step toward balancing your pH. Soda's extremely acid-forming nature contributes to headaches, pain disorders, and other symptoms of an acid-forming diet. If you're prone to headaches or pain, you'll notice pain levels will drop (after you're finished with any caffeine-withdrawal headaches, if you've been addicted to caffeine). If you don't have any pain disorders, you'll likely find that you're less prone to them later in life if you stop drinking soda now.

60-Second Weight-Loss Tip #6:
Learn to Limit Sugar

Sugar quickly converts to fat in your body. Eating less of it goes a long way toward helping you achieve your desired weight.

You've learned about the problems of aspartame and sucralose. But synthetic sweeteners are not the only ones that cause acidity and weight gain. Naturally occurring sugar is still one of the worst foods you can consume, particularly if you're trying to lose weight.

As you learned earlier, on average we eat over 2½ pounds of sugar weekly, which adds up to more than 150 pounds of sugar annually in the form of sugary soft drinks, sweetened juices, cookies, cakes, pastries, and processed and prepared foods. Compare that with what our ancestors ate a century ago: only 5 pounds of sugar annually.

Linked to high blood pressure, high cholesterol, heart disease, weight gain, diabetes, and premature aging—to name only a few—sugar in the amounts we consume is one of the worst substances we put into our bodies. Even a fairly small amount suppresses your immune system for between 4 and 6 hours, giving any viruses or bacteria you've been exposed to a heady advantage to take hold of your body. From ketchup and burgers to seasoning salts and juice, sugar may be lurking in the most unlikely places.

Here's the good news: Sugar consumption is easy to reduce because we are starting from such a high quantity.

How to Benefit

If you haven't already thrown out anything in your cupboards or fridge that contains sweetener, now is the time to do so. Look for any ingredient that contains -*ose*, such as glucose, high fructose corn syrup, dextrose, maltose, etc. Instead, use small amounts (a maximum of 1 teaspoon three times a day) of pure, unpasteurized honey, pure maple syrup, barley malt, agave nectar, or the herb stevia. Replacing sugar with most artificial sugar substitutes is like replacing one poison with another. If you're eating sugar substitutes, now is the time to kick the aspartame, lose the sucralose, and shun every food containing artificial sweeteners. No exceptions.

Stevia is the best choice and the only one that doesn't affect blood sugar levels. It is naturally between 300 and 1,000 times sweeter than sugar, depending on whether you're using the whole herb or the liquid extract. I find liquid stevia has the best taste and the least aftertaste. You can combine it with fresh juices like lemon or lime juice and water to make a delicious lemonade or limeade, or use it to sweeten hot or iced herbal teas. You can even use it when baking (although most recipes will need ingredient adjustments when using stevia). However, beware many powdered stevia products, which contain harmful additives or other sweeteners. Be sure to check labels before you buy.

Also, eliminate alcohol, since it is essentially just sugar.

Super Health Bonus

Even a few teaspoons of sugar at a time will suppress your immune system for 4 to 6 hours. Most cookies, pastries, pies, cakes, and other sweets contain far more sugar than that. By greatly reducing the amount of sugar you consume, you'll not only lose weight, but you'll also restore your immune system, becoming far less likely to succumb to whatever virus is "going around."

60-Second Weight-Loss Tip #7:
Eliminate Suspected Food Sensitivities

Common food sensitivities can cause bloating and weight gain.

When most people hear the term "food sensitivities," they imagine a stuffed or runny nose, itchy eyes, or other common symptoms from environmental allergens. While food sensitivities can cause these symptoms, they can also masquerade as other health issues, including weight gain and bloating.

Tissue swelling or bloating is a common symptom linked to eating foods to which you are sensitive. Some people lose weight just from cutting out those trigger foods. Some foods that commonly cause sensitivities are wheat, dairy products, corn and corn derivatives, soy, refined sugar, eggs, coffee or caffeine, beef, fish, or shellfish. Of course, there are others, but these are the most common offenders.

If you think this is a rare problem, you'll be surprised to learn that food sensitivities are on the rise. According to Ellen Cutler, DC, author of *The Food Allergy Cure*, an estimated 90 million people suffer from food allergies or sensitivities. I believe it is because more of our food supply has become genetically modified and tainted with pesticides and other synthetic ingredients during the growing or manufacturing processes. Our bodies are simply not designed to handle the onslaught of foreign substances we're throwing at them.

Genetic modification poses a particularly serious threat. Consider: If a nut protein is crossed with the soybean plant during the genetic engineering process, the soybean plant may now produce an allergic reaction in someone who is allergic to peanuts, putting that person at risk for anaphylactic shock or even death. Now, that is an extreme example, but the problem may be widespread when we're talking about food sensitivities, where many of the proteins used during genetic engineering are unknown, don't appear on product labels, and may elicit an unexpected response, including bloating and weight gain.

Another factor behind the rise in food sensitivities is the common use of certain foods. We discussed the weight gain linked to high fructose corn syrup (HFCS) earlier, but its rampant use is also causing corn to be a common culprit in food sensitivities. Overconsumption of any food or food ingredient can predispose the immune system for sensitivities and allergies.

Many food additives and artificial colors found in packaged, prepared, and fast foods are manufactured from coal tar or petroleum products. I jokingly tell my clients that these food additives are made from the petroleum products we can't put into our vehicles. But it's probably not far from the truth.

Most people crave the foods that they are sensitive to. It sounds contradictory, but it happens because of an allergic addiction that occurs. In the same way that a smoker may feel temporary improvement in his jitteriness and anxiety by smoking something as harmful as a cigarette, someone with food sensitivities may feel a temporary mood or physical uplift after eating a food to which she is sensitive. A craving for chocolate, for example, may indicate sensitivity to it.

As you balance your pH, you may also notice that sensitivities improve. This is because acidity in your body can make you susceptible to food sensitivities. Even seasonal allergies often subside or are greatly improved.

How to Benefit

While many people recommend rotation diets of specific foods and food families, that is simply not plausible for most people. If you suspect you are sensitive to a particular food, eliminate it from your diet for a month and see how you feel. It may take a while to notice an improvement because the food can still be in your system or causing inflammation in your body long after you last ingested it. If you suspect sensitivities, but are not sure what foods are the culprits, try eliminating the most common ones above. Most people feel tremendously better after doing so. Any excess weight comes off easier as well. If you constantly feel ill or have mysterious symptoms that nothing seems to help, you'd be wise to consult a natural health practitioner who specializes in food sensitivity testing. The skin-prick tests done by most allergists catch only severe food allergies, not sensitivities. Some practitioners use NAET (short for Nambudripad's Allergy Elimination Technique) or BioSET to identify sensitivities and help the body cope with these foods.

Super Health Bonus

If you eliminate foods to which you are sensitive, you'll experience much higher energy levels.

60-Second Weight-Loss Tip #8:
Don't Bother with Diet Pills

Diet pills contain the chemical phenylethylamine, which will make you binge once you stop taking them.

Most commercial diet products—particularly diet pills—do not work. Over-the-counter diet pills usually contain the ingredient phenylethyl-amine, which should be avoided. These pills trick your brain into thinking that you're not hungry, which may be fine while you're taking them. But as soon as you stop taking the pills and return to the generally unhealthy eating patterns most people have, you'll find the weight quickly returns. Or worse, you may gain more weight than you started with.[8]

How to Benefit

This is fairly straightforward. Just avoid or stop taking diet pills. Of course, if they are prescribed by your physician, you should consult her first.

Super Health Bonus

Not only will you avoid the rebound weight gain linked with diet pills, you'll also avoid the heartburn, nausea, constipation, headaches, and insomnia to which they are linked.

60-Second Weight-Loss Tip #9:
Don't Drink Diet Shakes

Glutamate, the protein that is found in most weight-loss drinks, can actually make you fatter.

Diet drinks are usually high-protein shakes made with isolated amino acids (amino acids are the building blocks of protein). Your body requires many different amino acids to build new tissue, heal existing tissue, and perform many other functions. A deficiency in just one can cause a host of health issues. Most diet drinks encourage amino acid deficiencies by using amino acids in a way not intended by nature.

Using certain synthetically derived amino acids like glutamine in an altered form such as glutamate can cause the body to have severe negative reactions such as headaches, weight gain, bloating, and edema, among other problems.

Diet shakes are not substitutes for a healthy diet. Having said that, replacing a meal with a highly nutritious shake can help with weight-loss efforts, provided you include the right ingredients and avoid the harmful ones. Use my Alkalizing Almond Milk (page 246) as a base for making your own smoothies, and add ground flaxseeds, green powder, and your favorite fruit, so you can forgo the store-bought diet shakes.

How to Benefit

Start by purchasing a whole foods protein powder. My favorite is pumpkin seed powder since it is not only a good source of protein but is also loaded with essential fats that help with weight loss and with the mineral zinc, which your body needs to keep your immune system strong and to build strong hair and nails, to name a few of its benefits.

While many people espouse whey protein, I'm not a fan. In my two decades of experience as a clinical nutritionist, I've seen countless people who are sensitive to dairy products. Whey is a derivative of dairy. In addition to being a common food allergen, dairy products, as you know from reviewing The Essential Plan, are acid forming and do more harm to your body than good. And since soy is also a common allergen, soy protein powders are best avoided as well.

Avoid any protein powders that contain isolated protein, isolated vegetable protein, or isolated soy protein, since these unnatural ingredients have been linked to many health issues. Additionally, avoid any protein powders that contain autolyzed or hydrolyzed ingredients since they usually reflect isolated proteins that are damaging to the body. Typically these ingredients indicate the presence of MSG, which you'll learn more about in 60-Second Weight-Loss Tip #10 on page 106.

Super Health Bonus

Not only will you notice that it's easier to lose weight when you eliminate diet shakes containing glutamate, you'll find that by avoiding the protein powders containing isolated amino acids, you'll have fewer headaches and other nagging health concerns.

60-Second Weight-Loss Tip #10:
Uncover Hidden MSG

This common food additive causes you to feel hungry even when you're not.

Protein powders and shakes are not the only hiding places for isolated amino acids. Anything that contains monosodium glutamate (MSG) is also an issue. And unfortunately, MSG has not only been shown in countless studies to be linked to weight gain and hunger, but it's also a proven neurotoxin—a toxin that does serious damage to the brain and nervous system.

According to Russell Blaylock, MD, MSG researcher, neurologist, and author of *Excitotoxins: The Taste that Kills*, here are some of the most common hiding places for MSG.

- **Soups.** Most soups, including homemade soups, contain MSG—even if the cook swears otherwise. That's because most soup bases, commercial stocks, and bouillon powder and cubes contain MSG. The best approach is to make your own soup stock. Simply chop onions, celery, and carrots, add leftover chicken bones, a teaspoon of apple cider vinegar to draw the alkaline calcium out of the bones (learn more about this technique in Tip #16 on page 125), and herbs such as bay leaves, basil, thyme, and rosemary, and let simmer for an hour or two in a large stockpot filled with water. You can make a vegetarian stock by omitting the bones.

- **Spice mixtures.** Love that Cajun seasoning, Tex-Mex rub, or other spice mixture? Most spice mixtures contain MSG—frequently in the form of autolyzed yeast or yeast extract. Choose organic spices and blend your own spice mixtures. My favorite is Harmonic Arts, which makes a variety of excellent spice mixtures.

- **Infant formula.** As terrible as it sounds, some brands of infant formula actually contain MSG in one of its myriad disguises (get the full list below).

- **Soy products.** Many of the vegetarian burgers, hot dogs, sausages, and other meat alternatives contain textured vegetable protein (TVP), hydrolyzed vegetable protein, or hydrolyzed plant protein, all of which usually contain MSG.

- **Baby food.** Shockingly, manufacturers of baby food often include glutamate—one of MSG's many guises—as a flavor "enhancer."

- **Bottled sauces.** Whether Thai, teriyaki, or Jamaican jerk sauce, most bottled sauces contain MSG.

- **Salad dressings.** Many store-bought salad dressings you use could be negating any of the health benefits of eating salad—that is, if you choose a bottled dressing that contains MSG. Bottled salad dressings may have "natural flavor," "spices," or "seasoning," all of which can legally contain MSG.

- **Salad croutons.** Most croutons are flavored with bouillon, soup base, or "natural" or artificial flavors that contain MSG.

- **Protein powders.** Many of the protein powders used for weight loss or muscle building—even those sold in health food stores—can contain MSG, usually in the form of hydrolyzed protein or hydrolyzed soy protein.

- **Vaccines.** Many vaccines contain MSG or glutamate. The chickenpox and the measles, mumps, and rubella (MMR) vaccines are two common examples.

MSG appears in many other forms—some of the most common ones are listed below—and none of them are good for you.

This dangerous additive can be found in flavors added to many foods and often is listed on labels as "natural flavor," "natural beef or chicken flavoring," or "natural flavoring."

This nervous system toxin masquerades in many other food additives. We've already talked about a number of them, but so you know what to look for on food labels, here is a list of additives that always contain MSG:[9]

- Autolyzed yeast
- Calcium caseinate
- Hydrolyzed oat flour
- Hydrolyzed plant protein
- Hydrolyzed protein
- Hydrolyzed vegetable protein
- Monosodium glutamate (that's the full name for MSG)

- Plant protein extract
- Sodium caseinate
- Textured protein
- Yeast extract

Additives that frequently contain MSG:
- Bouillon
- Broth
- Flavoring
- Malt extract
- Malt flavoring
- Natural beef or chicken flavoring
- Natural flavoring
- Seasoning
- Spices
- Stock

Additives that sometimes contain MSG:
- Carrageenan
- Enzymes
- Soy protein concentrate
- Soy protein isolate
- Whey protein isolate

How to Benefit

It's inexcusable, considering the volumes of research proving the damaging effects of MSG, that government agencies still allow the food-processing and fast-food industries to continue using this toxin. Until they stop, you need to take charge of the food ingredients that you're consuming. Next time you're buying packaged foods, be sure to take the above list with you to avoid harmful chemicals that are most likely sabotaging your weight-loss efforts and negatively impacting your health.

Super Health Bonus

Eliminating MSG from your diet can have innumerable effects in addition to weight loss. Because MSG is linked to mood disorders, headaches and migraines, anxiety disorders, attention deficit hyperactivity disorder (ADHD), depression, autism, and many others, you may notice that your moods become more balanced, your anxiety and depression diminish, you have fewer headaches and migraines, and your mental alertness improves.

60-Second Weight-Loss Tip #11:
Reduce Pesticides and Heavy Metals

Pesticides and heavy metals disrupt your body's natural fat-burning processes. Once you reduce your exposure, your body will be better able to rebalance.

Common toxins found in the environment, food, personal care products, and surprising other sources can interfere with your body's natural fat-burning processes by impairing important enzymes involved in metabolism. These harmful toxins include heavy metals and pesticides.[10]

Pesticides act as free radicals in the body. Free radicals have damaging effects in the body, including damaging cell walls that may use cholesterol buildup as a repair mechanism and disrupting the internal mechanisms of cells, which may lead to genetic damage or harm the cells' ability to function properly.

According to research compiled by the US Food and Drug Administration's Agricultural Marketing Service, Pesticide Data Program, today's apple contains the residue of many toxic chemicals used during the growing process. In just one category of chemicals known as organophosphate insecticides, this federal government agency found residue of 10 different neurotoxins: azinophos-methyl, chlorpyrifos, diazinon, dimethoate, ethion, omethoate, parathion, parathion-methyl, phosalone, and phosmet. The average apple is sprayed with pesticides 17 times before it is harvested. Many of these pesticides are hormone disruptors that throw off the delicate hormonal balance required for maintaining a healthy weight.

How to Benefit

Don't spray your lawn with pesticides. Avoid using pesticides or insecticides in your home. Choose organic produce as much as possible, particularly for the "dirty dozen." The dirty dozen are foods that research shows consistently contain high levels of pesticides. They are peaches, apples, bell peppers, celery, nectarines, strawberries, cherries, lettuce, grapes, pears, spinach, and potatoes. If you aren't able to purchase only organic products, be sure to try to find organic variations of the dirty dozen especially.

It's not possible to eliminate all metals from your body or your life. But you can make a difference in how they much they affect you by greatly reducing your exposure and taking measures to detoxify them from your body.

Super Health Bonus

By eliminating pesticides from your home and lawn you may decrease your risk of brain diseases like Parkinson's. Parkinson's disease has been linked to pesticide exposures by large amounts of research.

As for heavy metals, cadmium, lead, and mercury are toxic to the brain and nervous system. They are linked to dementia, Alzheimer's disease, learning disabilities, seizure disorders, aggression, hyperactivity, heart arrhythmias, headaches, and many other health issues. Reducing your exposure may reduce your chances of experiencing one of these disorders.

Here are some of the surprising sources of cadmium, lead, and mercury.

CADMIUM IS FOUND IN:

- Automobile seat covers
- Black rubber
- Burned motor oil
- Ceramics
- Cigarettes

- Evaporated milk
- Fertilizers
- Floor coverings
- Fungicides
- Furniture
- Refined wheat flour (white flour)
- Silver polish
- Soft drinks from vending machines with cadmium in the pipes

LEAD IS FOUND IN:

- Canned food
- Cigarette smoke (even secondhand smoke)
- Colored, glossy newsprint
- Some ceramic dishes
- Lead paint in older homes
- Lead water pipes in older buildings
- Refined chocolate
- Vehicle emissions (yes, even though lead gasoline was banned two decades ago in some countries)

MERCURY IS FOUND IN:

- Dental fillings that look silver (Many dentists cite studies that show no mercury particles have been released from fillings, but numerous studies show that mercury is primarily released as a vapor to gain access to the brain and blood.)
- Fish (not all fish, but many farmed varieties tend to be contaminated with mercury)
- Immunizations (Many vaccines, even those used for children, contain the mercury-based preservative thimerosol in excessive amounts.)

60-Second Weight-Loss Tip #12:
Wipe Out White Flour

This particular type of carb leads to weight gain and dangerous blood sugar spikes.

According to research by Katherine L. Tucker, PhD, of the Jean Mayer USDA Human Nutrition Research Center on Aging, Tufts University, people who eat three or four servings daily of foods made with white flour (including white bread, wheat bread, bagels, muffins, pancakes, cookies, pies, and cakes) have significantly larger waistlines than people whose carbs come primarily from whole grains.

That's not surprising when you understand that refined flour and the baked goods and cereals made from them are treated almost the same as white sugar in your body. They cause rapid blood sugar spikes, which cause your pancreas (the organ just below your ribs on the left side of your abdomen that regulates digestion and blood sugar) to secrete insulin. Insulin is necessary in small doses. But in large doses, like those dumped after eating white flour and white sugar–based foods, it signals your body to store fat. That stored fat can sit on your abdomen, but it can also be added to your hips, arms, butt, or other places on your body.

Conversely, research shows that when people stay on a high-protein, low-carb diet, they expend fewer and fewer calories during physical activity.[11] The longer they stay on the program, the worse it gets. So they need more exercise to lose weight the longer they stay on a low-carb diet. What's the solution? Avoid the wrong carbs and choose moderate amounts of the right ones.

How to Benefit

Avoid eating foods made with refined sugar or white or wheat flour. That list typically includes white bread, wheat bread, bagels, muffins, pancakes, waffles, cookies, pies, and cakes, though you can make healthy substitutions when baking your own. Over time your desire for these types of foods will diminish. If you're still craving sweets, eat a meal or a snack more often— about every 2 to 3 hours. Be sure your meal contains some protein foods like fish, chicken, nuts, seeds, tofu, or beans. Eating more healthy fats such as coconut oil, flaxseeds and flaxseed oil, avocado, and nuts can also help you feel full longer. You can also supplement with chromium.

Super Health Bonus

You'll experience more energy if you avoid these refined carbs. They may give you a short burst of energy, but they cause a major crash within an hour or two, causing you to crave more as a short-lived pick-me-up. This cycle takes its toll on your energy levels and your adrenal glands—the two triangular glands that sit on top of your kidneys and help you cope with stress of all kinds, from allergies and temperature changes to emotional stresses. Packing in the harmful carbs will take a load off of your adrenal glands and balance your blood sugar levels. You'll have more energy and balanced moods.

Also, eat moderate amounts of healthy carbs. They include most vegetables (sorry, potatoes don't work on a slimming program), whole grains, legumes, and fruit (eat fruit occasionally, and avoid pineapples and bananas until you've reached your target weight—and then eat them only in minimal amounts, because of the high amount of sugars they contain).

60-Second **SUCCESS STORY**

Sherrie Baker

Age: **46**
Location: **Elmira, ON, Canada**
Occupation: **Health kinesiologist**

Total Weight Lost:
13 pounds

Total Inches Lost:
9.25

"My skin is clearer, smoother, and younger looking."

How I Got Here:

Feeling "very overweight, sluggish, and constipated," Sherrie Baker was ready to try a new approach to weight loss. Other programs just didn't work for her, no matter how well she stuck with them. She admitted, "To be honest, I wasn't really putting much faith in 60 Seconds to Slim working." Then she thought to herself, "I didn't have anything to lose, and the question went through my mind:

What if it works?" That's when she decided to give my plan a fair try.

She had some obstacles to overcome, particularly bad habits such as not exercising and making poor food choices for the sake of convenience.

When I asked Sherrie about her goals, she said, "I honestly didn't expect the program to work, so I had very modest goals of maybe losing a few pounds."

Progress Report:

Sherrie experienced greater energy on the program and lost more weight and inches than she thought possible for her. She shared that she used to get terrible menstrual cramps and headaches but didn't experience those symptoms while on the program. She thought that the afternoon headaches she had every single day were just part of life, but they stopped altogether and she hasn't had one in several months. "I enjoyed the food immensely and after being on the program for a couple of weeks my food cravings completely changed," she told me.

"My skin is clearer, smoother, and younger looking, and many people have commented on that. When I began the diet, I had been having pain in my left breast for a month or two, and about a month into the program I decided to use health kinesiology to test what was going on. The conclusion was early breast cancer and the treatment was to continue with the eating plan I was on as well as some health kinesiology corrections that were necessary to help things along."

Beyond:

Sherrie is still following 60 Seconds to Slim. She says: "I can totally give credit to Michelle's eating plan as the major reason why I am now cancer free 3 months later. All testing at the breast clinic has given me a clean bill of health! I see this way of eating as something that I will do for the rest of my life. I have no desire to eat high-sugar, processed, or high-fat foods ever again. In fact, when I do cheat, I feel awful and realize how bad for my body non-whole foods really are. I also must say that I am fully convinced that the amount of water that is required on the program is also a huge contributor to the weight loss, lack of muscle aches, and generally feeling great overall. Thank you, Michelle, for doing the research to bring us such a wonderful eating plan that helps to restore health and balance in the body! I am definitely recommending it for my clients.

Chapter 4

Week 2: BOOST

Eat More of These Metabolism-Boosting Superfoods

In this section you will learn about some of the most important and proven fat-burning foods, why it is important to include them in your diet, the best ways to benefit from these foods, and how you can start eating more of them. Add at least five of these 60-Second Weight-Loss Tips this week—or more if you'd like—and continue eating these superfoods throughout the program. Each boosts your metabolism, burns fat, or detoxifies fat and eliminates inflammation. The one thing they have in common is that they all boost your body's ability to lose fat. Many of these foods are alkalizing. Those that aren't are what I call Wise Acid foods, since they have so many beneficial properties that they should still be a part of your diet.

Here are the 60-Second Weight-Loss Tips you'll learn this week. Choose at least five. Going forward, you may notice some duplication between tips.

13. Fire Up Fat Burning with Chiles (page 120)

Chiles charge your metabolism to burn more fat.

14. Add Garlic and Onions to Strengthen Your Liver (page 121)

Eating onions and garlic daily strengthens your liver and reduces your chances of being among the 65 percent of Americans who are at risk for nonalcoholic fatty liver disease and resulting weight gain.

15. Snack on Almonds (page 124)

Snacking on almonds increases weight loss by 64 percent and targets belly fat.

16. Choose Apple Cider Vinegar (page 125)

Simply choosing the right condiment can bolster your body's fat-digestion capabilities and reduce appetite.

17. Drink Green Tea (page 126)

Study after study proves that drinking green tea dramatically reduces weight.

18. Add Seaweed to Your Diet (page 127)

The fiber found in seaweed keeps you feeling full longer so you'll need less food and burn more fat.

19. Cook with Coconut Oil (page 129)

Cooking with coconut oil helps to reset the thyroid gland to turn up the heat on your metabolism.

20. Add More Raw Foods (page 131)

Enzymes found in raw foods are natural fat burners, yet 80 percent of people don't get enough in their diets.

21. Eat Omega-3 Fats Before Working Out (page 135)

Omega-3 fatty acids fire up belly fat loss during workouts when consumed within an hour of exercising.

22. Choose Complex Carbs (page 136)

Complex carbs balance your body chemistry to speed fat loss.

23. Season Your Food with the Top Five Fat-Burning Spices (page 137)

Add the Top Five Fat-Burning Spices to your diet to ramp up your weight loss.

24. Eat the Top Five Fat-Burning Fruits (page 138)

Adding more of these surprising fruits to your diet speeds fat loss.

25. Eat the Top Five Nuts, Seeds, and Oils (page 140)

These five nuts, seeds, and oils help your body to burn more fat.

26. Eat Five More Foods That Burn Fat (page 141)

Add these five foods and beverages to maximize fat loss.

27. Eat Red, Purple, and Black Foods (page 143)

The antioxidant anthocyanin causes dramatic weight loss and is found in dark and reddish foods like red or purple grapes, black beans, beets, cherries, and more.

28. Drink Water with Lemon Juice (page 144)

Drinking plenty of water with fresh lemon juice helps to flush toxins from fat cells.

29. Get Enough Ellagic Acid (page 145)

When eaten in moderate amounts, the powerful nutrient found in many fruits, particularly cherries, grapes, and berries, supercharges the liver's ability to break down hormones and toxins and burn fat.

30. Eat Cruciferous Vegetables and Leafy Greens (page 146)

Cruciferous vegetables and leafy greens contain a potent compound that stops your body from storing fat while helping to eliminate toxins.

31. Enjoy Grapefruit Daily (page 147)

When grapefruit is eaten on a daily basis, it can cause you to lose up to 20 pounds in 13 weeks.

32. Replenish Bowel Flora (page 148)

Adding critical bacteria to your diet can dramatically boost your weight-loss efforts by restoring bowel health and eliminating infections.

33. Add Sprouts to Your Meals (page 151)

Sprouts significantly boost fat loss and rev up your energy—with almost no calories.

34. Add the Ancient Grain Quinoa to Your Diet (page 158)

Quinoa is a fat-busting superfood that helps you balance blood sugar and lose weight.

60-Second Weight-Loss Tip #13:
Fire Up Fat Burning with Chiles

Chiles charge your metabolism to burn more fat.

If you've ever eaten spicy food, chances are that you are familiar with capsaicin. It is the phytonutrient found in chiles that turns up the heat in a meal and has the added benefit of stoking your fat-burning furnace. If you've noticed you've broken out in a sweat after eating a bowl of curry or another dish with chiles, that's a sign that the capsaicin has kicked your metabolism up a few notches.

Capsaicin is naturally found in chile peppers of all kinds, from poblanos to jalapeños, banana peppers to habaneros. According to research in the *American Journal of Clinical Nutrition*, its heat reduces excess insulin in the body by speeding metabolism and lowering blood sugar to healthy levels before excess insulin can signal your body to store fat.[1]

In this study, people who were fed a meal containing a ground red pepper–chile blend had lower levels of insulin in their blood after eating than those who didn't eat the blend. Even more exciting, the more overweight people were, the better the results.

Canadian research published in the *British Journal of Nutrition* showed that capsaicin reduces hunger to the tune of about 200 fewer calories consumed each day.[2] It also is estimated to bolster the metabolism by 25 percent. Additionally, capsaicin is a natural anti-inflammatory that helps to take down the heat and inflammation linked to excess acidity, which, as you've learned, is linked with excess weight. So capsaicin is a real gem for anyone looking to shed some weight. (You'll learn more about other fat-burning spices in Tip #23 on page 137.)

How to Benefit

Choose fresh, frozen, or cooked chiles since the active ingredient, capsaicin, is still intact in these forms. Research shows that capsaicin's ability to speed metabolism drops by 23 percent when chiles have been dried and turned into powder. Simply add chopped chile peppers to your soups, stews, and curries. You can also chop and add them to a small amount of coconut oil to create a spicy sandwich spread or cooking oil. Of course, store the chile oil covered in the refrigerator; it will last for about a week. Alternatively, you can use a nasal spray called Sinus Buster that also provides the benefits of capsaicin. One word of caution: It's hot. Your nasal and sinus cavities may burn for about a minute after using it, but it quickly dissipates after that.

Safety Consideration

Wear gloves when chopping particularly hot varieties of chiles. Avoid rubbing your eyes or touching your face after chopping them. Also, wash your hands thoroughly after touching them. I throw them into a small food processor to avoid chopping the hottest chiles by hand. Contrary to popular belief, chiles do not cause digestive troubles, burn the stomach, or cause ulcers. While they can aggravate existing ulcers and hemorrhoids, they are safe and soothing to the digestive tracts of most people.

Super Health Bonus

Research shows that capsaicin can effectively improve circulation and reduce pain and is particularly effective for arthritic symptoms.[3] Consuming capsaicin also causes a release of the feel-good hormones called endorphins, helping to boost mood and energy levels, so you can expect to have less pain and improved moods and energy. If you use the nasal spray, you'll likely notice improved breathing, reduced nasal inflammation, and less sinusitis if you suffer from the condition. Research also shows that capsaicin helps to protect against cancer by killing off abnormal cells before they can become cancerous.

60-Second Weight-Loss Tip #14:
Add Garlic and Onions to Strengthen Your Liver

Eating onions and garlic daily strengthens your liver and reduces your chances of being among the 65 percent of Americans who are at risk for nonalcoholic fatty liver disease and resulting weight gain.

The liver serves over 500 functions in the human body, making it one of our most overworked organs—particularly thanks to our modern lifestyle replete with a high-fat, high-sugar diet loaded with artificial preservatives, colors, and additives, along with pollutants in the air, soil, and water. The liver is the primary organ responsible for detoxifying all of these substances, along with all medications. So you can see how the liver is an essential organ that may need some support to maintain its heavy workload.

A high-sugar and high-fat diet also puts your liver at risk of becoming fatty. You may have heard of someone having a fatty liver.

Fatty liver is also known as nonalcoholic steatohepatitis (NASH) or nonalcoholic fatty liver disease (NAFLD). This is when the liver contains an excessive amount of fat that slowly replaces healthy liver tissue. When this happens, the liver becomes slightly enlarged and heavier. Fatty liver is a common problem, particularly in people who are overweight and over age 30.

Here are some signs you might have a fatty liver:

• You are overweight, particularly in the abdomen.

• You find it very hard to lose weight.

• You may have type 2 diabetes.

• You may feel exhausted.

• You may have a compromised immune system or experience frequent infections or colds or flu.

• You may have elevated triglycerides or cholesterol in your blood.

• You may have been diagnosed with syndrome X.[4]

It is not necessary to have all the symptoms above, or even to have any of the symptoms at all, to have a fatty liver. You should always consult your doctor if you suspect you may have any liver condition. Fortunately, the liver is a highly resilient organ. When fatty liver disease is caught early enough, there are many excellent ways to help reverse or to simply improve liver functioning. Here are some of my favorite ways to improve liver function.

• Supplement with liver-boosting herbs like those outlined in Tip #65 on page 227.

• Avoid trans and hydrogenated fats (read the labels)—you should be doing that already as part of The Essential Plan.

• Avoid fried foods.

- Switch to extra virgin olive oil or coconut oil for cooking (don't allow it to smoke).
- Eat a diet high in nonstarchy vegetables.

While all of these recommendations will help, one of the easiest and best things you can do is to eat more onions and garlic.

Garlic and onions contain sulfur compounds that increase the liver's ability to detoxify fat and harmful toxins. Once known as "Russian penicillin" for its effectiveness against strep, staph, and other bacteria, garlic is also powerful against many fungi and species of yeasts. Its combination of anti-infectious agents and detoxification-assisting compounds may be why it is able to help normalize liver function when eaten regularly.

Additionally, scientists believe that a compound found in garlic, prostaglandin A, may be the effective ingredient that inhibits harmful liver enzymes and improves the way fats are metabolized in the liver. You'll learn more about other spices that burn fat in Tip #23 on page 137.

How to Benefit

Eat at least one clove of garlic daily, preferably raw. This is easy to do when you make my Super Fat-Burning Salsa (see page 255) and enjoy it with vegetable crudités. You can also stir freshly minced garlic into your soup, stew, curry, or tomato sauce just before serving. Another idea: Add a clove of raw garlic to your salad dressings. I have a few dressing recipes to help you out, beginning on page 266. Or cut a small amount off the top of a whole head of garlic, drizzle with a small amount of olive oil, cover in a baking dish, and bake in a 300°F oven for about 45 minutes to enjoy a delicious garlic-buttery type of spread.

Super Health Benefit

According to scientists at the New York University Medical Center and the University of Texas System Cancer Center, serious garlic eaters have a reduced risk of colon and stomach cancer.[5] You'll also be supercharging your liver while warding off cancer. That's better than any liver drug can offer.

60-Second Weight-Loss Tip #15:
Snack on Almonds

Snacking on almonds increases weight loss by 64 percent and targets belly fat.

Did you know that there is a no-cook, no-fuss snack that you can eat throughout the day that is not only tasty but also shrinks belly fat? In a study conducted at California's City of Hope National Medical Center and published in the *International Journal of Obesity and Related Metabolic Disorders*, overweight participants who snacked on 70 almonds daily had a 14 percent waistline reduction.[6] Of course, they were following a healthful diet along with eating the almonds throughout the day, and by following the 60 Seconds to Slim Plan, you will be making healthier choices like this one that have the potential to add up!

According to researchers, almonds turn on feelings of fullness and satiety, causing people to feel less hungry and eat less.

When eaten in small amounts every 3 hours, almonds help keep blood sugar levels stable. And stable blood sugar levels not only help keep you feeling full longer; they also stop your body from pumping out hormones that tell your body to hoard fat. Additionally, almonds are rich in calcium—a mineral that has been proven to help speed up weight-loss efforts as well as to be essential in regulating your body's pH.

How to Benefit

Enjoy unsweetened almond milk in place of cow's milk when you bake, on your cereal, in smoothies, or on its own. Snack on raw, unsalted almonds throughout the day to keep your blood sugar levels stable and cause your body to release fat from its stores. Even better: Soak the almonds overnight in some pure water, then drain and snack on the hydrated, plumped-up almonds throughout the day. This simple soaking process can dramatically improve nutrition content and digestibility. I usually recommend eating 10 almonds every 2 hours to help regulate blood sugar levels and significantly help with weight loss. Stop snacking at least 2 to 3 hours before bedtime.

Super Health Bonus

The calcium in almonds helps build and maintain strong teeth, nails, blood, skin, and soft tissues. It is essential to our brain's ability to connect with our body via proper nerve signals. Additionally, it helps relax our nerves, allowing us to better cope with stress. Almonds are also high in magnesium, which is vitally important to our health and well-being. It is involved in producing energy for most of our bodily processes and even in structuring our basic genetic material. Almonds are also high in protein and fiber and are a good source of B-complex vitamins, vitamin E, and iron. They help to increase energy and balance moods, and they are the perfect antistress food when eaten on a regular basis. Their fiber content binds to toxins in your body to help you detox.

60-Second Weight-Loss Tip #16:
Choose Apple Cider Vinegar

Simply choosing the right condiment can bolster your body's fat-digestion capabilities and reduce appetite.

According to nutrition researcher Larrian Gillespie, MD, when a group of women were asked to add 1½ tablespoons of apple cider vinegar to their salad at lunch, they ate 200 fewer calories at their next meal.[7] Apple cider vinegar may slow the digestion and absorption of starches, causing people to feel full longer.

Keep in mind that apple cider vinegar is a Wise Acid, so you'll need to balance out the acidity with lots of salad greens and other vegetables to keep your pH on the alkaline side of the spectrum. And the myth that apple cider vinegar has an alkalizing effect on your body after it's ingested is just that: a myth.

How to Benefit

Add apple cider vinegar to extra virgin olive oil and a clove of raw garlic for a delicious and fast salad dressing. Toss with salad greens. Alternatively, drink a teaspoon of apple cider vinegar mixed with ½ cup of water about 30 minutes prior to eating each meal and you'll feel fuller but experience less indigestion and bloating.

Super Health Bonus

Apple cider vinegar contains malic and tartaric acids, which help break down fats and proteins in the stomach. You may find you're feeling less bloated after a meal. Additionally, malic acid has been proven to reduce fibromyalgia pain. Apple cider vinegar also helps kill urinary tract infections.

60-Second Weight-Loss Tip #17:
Drink Green Tea

Study after study proves that drinking green tea dramatically reduces weight.

Green tea is a fat buster extraordinaire. It contains the phytonutrient epigallocatechin gallate (or EGCG for short). EGCG has been proven in multiple studies to increase the rate at which fat is burned in your body.

Multiple studies also show that green tea targets belly fat. Research at Tufts University indicates that EGCG in green tea, like other catechins, activates fat-burning genes in the abdomen to speed weight loss by 77 percent. New research published in the *Journal of Nutrition* found that overweight adults who drank 4 to 6 cups of green tea daily lost at least 7 percent more abdominal fat than those who didn't drink green tea.

As if that wasn't enough reason for most of us to include foods high in catechins like green and white tea in our diet, catechins also improve your body's ability to use insulin secreted by your pancreas, which prevents blood sugar spikes and crashes involved in plummeting energy levels, depression, mood swings, fatigue, irritability, and cravings for unhealthy foods.

How to Benefit

Add 1 or 2 teaspoons of green tea leaves to a cup of boiling water, preferably in a tea strainer. Let steep for 5 minutes. Pour over ice if you prefer a cold beverage. Alternatively, use a quality green tea in tea bag form for convenience. One tea bag should equal about 1 teaspoon of green tea. Avoid the green tea–based flavored tea bags or premade beverages unless you are certain that the "natural flavors" are MSG free. Bottled drinks are usually loaded with high fructose corn syrup or other sugars that more than negate any health benefits of drinking green tea.

Most experts recommend drinking at least 3 cups daily to obtain green tea's fat-burning benefits. And don't worry—it contains a lot less caffeine than coffee or black tea. If you're not wild about the flavor, try a few different kinds. Try it iced or hot. Add some of the natural herb stevia to sweeten it if you want a sweeter drink. I wasn't crazy about green tea the first few times I tried it, but now I love it with a fresh squeeze of lemon and a few drops of stevia over ice—voilà! See my recipe for Super Fat-Busting Green Tea Lemonade on page 245. Green tea is an acidic food, but it is a Wise Acid. By adding flavorless pH drops, you'll balance out some of the acidity without losing any of the health or weight-loss benefits of green tea.

Super Health Bonus

Research shows green tea may be helpful against a number of different cancer types. In an April 2010 study published in *Cancer Prevention Research*, EGCG was found to suppress lung cancer cell growth. In numerous other studies, EGCG appears to inhibit colorectal cancers. A March 2010 study in *Cancer Science* indicated that EGCG aids the body by causing prostate cancer cells to commit suicide. This catechin may prevent skin damage and wrinkling too. EGCG appears to be 200 times more powerful than vitamin E at destroying skin-damaging free radicals.[8] Free radicals react with healthy cells in the body and cause damage, so lessening their numbers may help reduce wrinkling and other signs of aging. Free radicals are increasingly linked to many serious chronic illnesses like arthritis, diabetes, and cancer. Because it is a potent antioxidant, EGCG can positively impact a lot more than just skin cells.

60-Second Weight-Loss Tip #18:
Add Seaweed to Your Diet

The fiber found in seaweed keeps you feeling full longer so you'll eat less food and burn more fat.

Scientist Morten Georg Jensen at the University of Copenhagen in Denmark found that alginate, a type of fiber found in brown seaweed, can help people lose weight when consumed regularly.[9] He studied the effects of different doses over 3 years and determined that people who drank fiber drinks with alginates ate less and felt less hungry.

In a 12-week study, Dr. Jensen followed 96 overweight men and women who drank a beverage containing alginate or a placebo on a daily basis. Participants who drank the seaweed fiber lost almost 4 pounds more on average, due to a decrease in body fat, than those who had the placebo.

Dr. Jensen concluded that the alginate may form a gel in the stomach that increases signals to the brain that a person is full.

How to Benefit

While the study was conducted with brown seaweed, all seaweed contains alginate, so you can choose the ones you like the most. There are many excellent types of seaweed. Even if you can't stand the taste of seaweed, you can benefit from eating it. Just select the varieties that don't have a seaweed-type taste, like agar agar—a natural gelling agent. I use it with fruit juice to make gelatin-like desserts with far more nutrition.

Or you can choose kelp noodles, which don't carry the high-carb problem linked to most pastas. You can eat kelp noodles every day and you won't get fat on them. You can make wraps from nori seaweed, or make a type of sushi with cooked and cooled quinoa and veggies rolled in nori sheets. Add dulse, kelp, arame, or other types of seaweed to soups and stews to benefit from their nutrition.

Be sure to eat the seaweed to get the benefit from the alginate—you won't get your fiber from a seaweed wrap at the spa. Most health food stores contain a wide variety of dried seaweed that is easy to reconstitute in water. Follow package instructions for each. Try to eat some seaweed every day for best results.

Super Health Bonus

Not only does seaweed help keep you feeling full longer, but its rich iodine content also helps to reboot your thyroid gland to further boost your metabolism when you make seaweed a part of your diet. Your thyroid gland cannot manufacture the hormones that control the rate of your metabolism without a sufficient supply of iodine. Adding iodine-rich seaweed is the perfect way to reset your thyroid gland, address possible nutrient deficiencies, and speed your metabolism. Check out 60-Second Weight-Loss Tip #19 on the facing page for another way to reset your thyroid!

60-Second Weight-Loss Tip #19:
Cook with Coconut Oil

Cooking with coconut oil helps to reset the thyroid gland to turn up the heat on your metabolism.

Simply switching your cooking oil can have a dramatic effect on your weight. It sounds too good to be true, but increasing amounts of research show that cooking with coconut oil can kick-start a sluggish thyroid gland. Here's why it works.

Your thyroid gland, the butterfly-shaped gland in the front of your neck, is the body's thermostat and helps to regulate the rate of metabolism, which is the rate of chemical processes that control the body's functions. Yet many people's thyroid glands are underactive, even when medical tests show normal functioning. According to some experts, as much as 25 percent of women may be affected by a sluggish thyroid gland.

When the thyroid gland is functioning poorly, it causes the rate of metabolism in our bodies to drop—sometimes significantly. This can happen because of stress, illness, hormonal fluctuations, and many other factors. Regardless of the cause, the effect is to slow down the rate at which our bodies turn food into energy, resulting in weight gain and fatigue.

It is certainly beneficial to have your thyroid function tested, especially if your difficulty losing weight has been accompanied by other symptoms of low thyroid function, including fatigue, feeling cold most of the time, poor memory or concentration, dry or flaky skin, headaches, mood swings, depression, hair loss, constipation, insomnia, and high cholesterol levels. You don't need to have all of these symptoms to have a low-functioning thyroid gland.

While blood tests can be beneficial, it is important to remember that most blood tests for thyroid gland function fail to catch a sluggish thyroid. Even if the tests do show abnormal results, in many cases thyroid medication does little to help with the excess weight and fatigue that many people with low thyroid function experience.

But it's not all bad news. Actually, whether you test positive for an underactive thyroid gland (known as hypothyroidism) or not, you can benefit from a simple dietary tweak that can reset your gland without any harmful side effects. The only side effects are that you may start to feel better than ever, lose weight, and have more energy.

That's where coconut oil comes in. Coconut oil researcher Bruce Fife, ND, found that regular consumption of coconut oil reverses hypothyroid gland problems and restores a slowed metabolism by stimulating thyroid hormones.[10] Research at the University of Colorado supports his findings. Scientists there found that coconut oil can increase calorie-burning power by up to 50 percent.

Coconut oil contains medium-chain tryglycerides (MCTs), a type of fatty acid that is easy to digest, stimulates the body's metabolism, and restores some of the body's natural enzyme activities needed to restore a healthy weight. Most other oils typically contain long-chain fatty acids, which can mean a significant difference to your body's metabolism and digestive functions, since these oils are harder to break down than those in coconut oil.

How to Benefit

Dr. Fife's research showed that 3 tablespoons of coconut oil daily can normalize low thyroid gland function.

Coconut oil is the best source of thyroid-resetting medium-chain triglycerides, but you can also obtain these fatty acids from coconut milk (full fat, not low fat), unsweetened shredded coconut, and fresh coconut. It takes about 7 ounces of fresh coconut (about half a coconut) or 2¾ cups (10 ounces, or 300 milliliters) of coconut milk per day to equal the desired 3½ tablespoons of coconut oil. Coconut rates as one of my Top Five Fat-Burning Fruits in Tip #24 (see page 138).

As a general rule, 3 ounces, or 88 milliliters, of coconut milk (not the low-fat variety) contains about 1 tablespoon of coconut oil. Try to get at least 3 tablespoons of coconut oil daily. It's easy when you sauté vegetables, poultry, fish, or other foods in coconut oil or coconut milk. You can stir a tablespoon of the oil into a smoothie or make your protein smoothie with coconut milk. I also bake with coconut oil. In most cases, you can replace margarine, butter, shortening, lard, or vegetable oil with the same amount of coconut oil in baking recipes. Coconut oil is used in most of the recipes at the back of this book, so if you need some inspiration to get started, check them out.

Super Health Bonus

In addition to the weight-loss benefits, eating a diet rich in medium-chain triglycerides has many other health benefits, including supporting your immune system and keeping your skin healthy looking. Additionally, MCTs are an excellent source of energy for the body and many people begin to feel more energetic when ingesting coconut oil on a daily basis. Medium-chain triglycerides also promote heart health. The Trobriand Islanders, who eat a high percentage of their daily diet in the form of coconuts, are virtually free of heart disease and atherosclerosis (not to mention obesity).

60-Second Weight-Loss Tip #20:
Add More Raw Foods

Enzymes found in raw foods are natural fat burners, yet 80 percent of people don't get enough in their diets.

Most people are deficient in an important nutritional factor that may be contributing to obesity and weight issues as well as low energy levels and other health conditions. Some experts estimate that 80 percent of people don't obtain sufficient enzymes in their diet.

You may not have even heard of enzymes. If you have, you may know that they aid digestion—but that is only the tip of the iceberg. Before I explain their role in weight loss, let me first review what enzymes are.

Enzymes are a specific type of protein that functions as the catalyst of every chemical reaction in your body. They affect every single life function, including thousands of essential biochemical reactions in the body and those that control excess weight. Every enzyme has a specialized function. Some enzymes control your body's ability to detoxify specific chemicals you breathe in from the air; others metabolize cholesterol and help eliminate excess amounts from the body. Some aid the digestion of specific components of food like proteins, carbohydrates, or fats.

While there are more than 5,000 known enzymes and potentially thousands more still undiscovered, they fall into three main categories: digestive, metabolic, and food enzymes. Some enzymes fall into more than one category, but I'll get to that momentarily.

Digestive enzymes assist your body in breaking down foods into their component nutrients so they can be properly absorbed. For example, the enzyme protease breaks protein foods down into the amino acids that compose proteins. The enzyme lipase breaks down fats in foods into fatty acids.

Metabolic enzymes are essential to properly run all of your body's biochemical processes, including breathing, thinking, moving, detoxifying, and healing. Each one serves a particular function not served by other enzymes. A deficiency in any metabolic enzyme can have catastrophic effects and be the basis for any number of serious medical conditions.

Food enzymes are found in raw foods like fruits, vegetables, sprouts, and herbs. These enzymes are destroyed by modern food processing and heating techniques, including canning, drying, packaging, microwaving, cooking, and others. While enzymes' role has been misunderstood for many years, leading scientists and researchers are beginning to prove that the more enzyme-depleted foods we eat, the faster we lose our internal supplies, resulting in weight gain, exhaustion, accelerated aging, and the onset of illness.

Prominent enzyme researcher Ellen Cutler, DC, indicates that about 80 percent of Americans get almost no enzymes in their diet. According to research by one of the earliest enzymologists, Edward Howell, MD, enzyme shortages are commonly seen in people suffering from obesity and many other health conditions.[11]

In an interview, Joseph Brasco, MD, a gastroenterologist at the Center for Colon and Digestive Disease in Huntsville, Alabama, stated: "Because the pancreas and liver need energy to produce enzymes, the resulting drain renders these organs temporarily unable to perform their functions of detoxification, blood sugar control, and fat burning."[12] All of these functions are essential for healthy weight management.

Exciting clinical data collected by Hiromi Shinya, MD, clinical professor of surgery at Albert Einstein College of Medicine, shows a correlation between the levels of enzymes in people's diets and the amounts of bodily enzymes they have.[13] This might not sound like a big deal, but it's huge.

Prior to his research, most mainstream doctors simply believed that the amount of enzymes in a person's diet had *no* link to the number of enzymes available for metabolic functions. But Dr. Shinya has shown that this popular misconception is wrong. His groundbreaking research has huge potential for anyone looking to lose weight or overcome disease, since many metabolic enzyme shortfalls are linked to impaired metabolic functions in the body.

So the good news is that by eating a diet high in enzyme-rich foods, we can improve the processes of metabolism, leading to weight loss and improved energy levels. Additionally, by supplementing with enzymes, we can improve our body's digestion and nutrient absorption. Further, by supplementing with enzymes on an empty stomach, we can dramatically promote health and the healing of specific functions in the body, including breaking down fat stores, detoxification, and the ability of the pancreas to balance blood sugar. I'll discuss the value of supplementing with enzymes and enzyme-packed sprouts later in this book. For now, let's get started with eating a diet higher in enzyme-rich food.

To counter the depletion of enzymes in our food and body we need to ingest more enzymes through food. Think of the balance between the need for enzymes, the depletion of enzymes, and the replenishing of enzymes through food as our "enzyme account." As with a bank account, if we always withdraw and never make deposits, we will eventually deplete our resources.

It is easy to add more enzyme-rich foods to your diet. Here are some simple ideas: Eat a large green salad as part of your lunch or dinner. Add some grated carrot, beetroot, or sprouts to your salads, sandwiches, or wraps. And eat soaked almonds as a protein- and fiber-packed snack throughout the day.

One of the best ways to obtain more enzymes is to add sprouts to your diet. Sprouts are packed with healing enzymes that can dramatically improve health. While it is not essential to eat sprouts on the 60 Seconds to Slim program, they are such nutrition powerhouses that you'll probably want to include them in your diet. In addition to being loaded with enzymes, they also contain high-quality protein, which increases during the sprouting process. The fiber content is usually quite high and increases during sprouting, and fiber helps balance blood sugar levels, keep us feeling full longer, and detoxify harmful substances that might otherwise find their way into fat stores in our bodies. The amounts of essential fatty acids, which we need for healthy weight management, also increase during the sprouting process.

Vitamin content, particularly vitamins A, C, E, and the B-complex vitamins, also increases during sprouting. The vitamin content of some seeds, grains, and beans can multiply by up to 20 times their original value within a few days of sprouting. Research shows that the sprouting process increases vitamin B_1 by up to 285 percent, vitamin B_2 by up to 515 percent, and niacin by up to 256 percent. You'll learn more in Tip #33 on page 151.

How to Benefit

Sprouts are so easy to add to your diet. Here are some ways to help you get started.

- Add a handful to your favorite salad recipe.
- Throw a large handful of mung bean sprouts into your favorite dish or stir-fry after you've removed it from the heat and are ready to serve it.
- Add alfalfa or clover sprouts to a sandwich or wrap.
- If you want to spice up a salad or sandwich, add some mustard, radish, or fenugreek sprouts for instant flavor.
- Mung bean sprouts make a delicious salad alongside your favorite veggies.

And, of course, always make sure you wash sprouts thoroughly before eating them.

Check out Simple Sprouting on page 154 if you'd like to grow your own. It's not a requirement on the 60 Seconds to Slim program, but it's a great addition to ramping up your weight-loss and energy effects. Ideally, try to make at least half of every meal and snack raw foods or sprouts.

Super Health Bonus

If your energy is waning and you want to experience greater vitality, add more enzyme-rich raw foods to your diet. Enzyme-rich foods don't give you the huge energy boosts and resulting energy crashes linked to stimulants. They gradually improve the functioning of your digestive system, liver, and pancreas, freeing energy from these functions and boosting cellular energy. Over days or weeks, you'll experience a serious energy boost. Most people report substantially more energy after a few days or weeks of eating more raw foods such as sprouts.

60-Second Weight-Loss Tip #21:
Eat Omega-3 Fats Before Working Out

Omega-3 fatty acids fire up belly fat loss during workouts when consumed within an hour before exercise.

You may have heard that omega-3 fatty acids are good for you. You may even know that they help with weight loss. But did you know that *when* you eat them plays a role in how much fat you'll burn? It's true.

Research shows that eating the right amount of these fats within 1 hour of working out will cause your body to burn 14 percent more fat than exercise alone.[14]

How to Benefit

Aim to eat a serving of fatty fish three times a week. Wild salmon, flounder, catfish, sardines, mackerel, herring, kipper, or whitebait are all great options. Tuna is also high in omega-3s, but limit how often you enjoy tuna if you are concerned about its high levels of mercury.

Enjoying a serving of fish just prior to your workout may not always be possible. And if you don't like fish, here are some great options to keep in mind:

- Eat a handful of raw, unsalted walnuts daily.
- Or, take 1 tablespoon of freshly ground flaxseeds twice daily.
- Or, take a daily fish oil supplement that contains 2,000 milligrams of eicosapentaenoic acid (EPA) and docosahexaenoic acid (DHA).

Eat the fish, flaxseeds, or walnuts or take the supplement within 1 hour of working out to speed fat loss.

Super Health Bonus

Omega-3 fatty acids also quell inflammation and pain in the body, so you may notice that your joints are freer and any pain you've experienced lessens too. Modern research is linking many chronic diseases for inflammation in the body. So, eating more inflammation-taming omega-3–rich foods will help you fend off countless diseases. You'll reduce your chances of experiencing diabetes, heart disease, brain disorders such as Alzheimer's disease, and more.

60-Second Weight-Loss Tip #22:
Choose Complex Carbs

Complex carbs balance your body chemistry to speed fat loss.

As you learned in Tip #12 on page 112, avoiding carbs can actually cause your body to start requiring more intense workouts just to get the same results as you initially had on a low-carb plan. So avoiding carbs is not the answer to long-term weight loss. By now you've eliminated the wrong carbs (the refined ones). So it's time to boost your metabolism by eating the right carbs in moderate amounts. No, that doesn't mean a plate piled high with pasta.

The right carbs are the ones that take a long time to digest. Simple or refined carbs are digested quickly and cause massive blood sugar spikes. Conversely, complex carbohydrates like whole grains, beans, nuts, and seeds take longer to digest, keep you feeling full longer, and help to ensure your body has the fuel it needs to create adequate amounts of feel-good hormones like serotonin. That's why depriving the body of carbs altogether often causes people to be irritable, depressed, or moody.

Not all complex carbs are alkalizing, though. It may take some time to get used to eating them, but there are many good alkalizing grains, nuts, seeds, and beans. It's not necessary to focus exclusively on these foods, but it does make keeping your pH alkaline easier. You can still enjoy smaller amounts of the Wise Acid grains, fruits, beans, nuts, and seeds. For a chart categorizing the pH of these foods, consult page 42.

How to Benefit

Carbs in the form of quinoa, spelt grains or 100 percent spelt flour foods, buckwheat groats or foods made with 100 percent buckwheat flour are excellent whole grain choices that are also alkalizing to your body. Unsalted soy nuts, edamame (green soybeans), lima beans, navy beans, lentils, tofu, and soy flour products are also alkalizing complex carbohydrates that are excellent choices. And pumpkin seeds, almonds, and sesame seeds are more alkalizing complex carbs that are great choices on the 60 Seconds to Slim Plan. See Tip #34 on page 158 for more information on quinoa.

Not all complex carbs are alkalizing. Some, like whole grain wheat, are actually quite acidic and not recommended on the program. Other good, albeit mildly to moderately acidic, choices include black beans, chickpeas, kidney beans, amaranth (a whole grain), kasha (buckwheat grains), millet (grain), triticale (grain), brown rice, wild rice, whole oats (oat bran is very acid forming and not a good choice), and 100 percent whole rye bread. These are Wise Acid Choices.

Occasional fruit snacks are fine as well. But remember that they are Wise Acid choices that should remain small components of your overall plan.

Super Health Bonus

By including alkalizing whole grains, legumes, nuts, and seeds in your diet you'll not only feel full longer, but you'll also maintain stable moods and reduce the likelihood of experiencing depression, since these foods provide the building blocks of feel-good hormones like serotonin.

60-Second Weight-Loss Tip #23:
Season Your Food with the Top Five Fat-Burning Spices

Add the top five fat-burning spices to your diet to ramp up your weight loss.

Losing weight can be as simple as spicing up your food. Use the following Top Five Fat-Burning Spices liberally in your recipes and cooking creations.

Garlic and onions: These yummy foods contain phytochemicals that break down fatty deposits in the body while also breaking down cholesterol; kill viruses, bacteria, and fungi; and protect against heart disease.[15] For more information, consult Tip #14 on page 121.

Turmeric: This popular spice, used primarily in Indian cooking, is the highest known source of beta-carotene, the antioxidant that helps protect the liver from free radical damage. Turmeric also helps your liver heal (see below) while helping your body metabolize fats by decreasing the fat storage rate in liver cells.[16]

Cinnamon: Researchers at the United States Department of Agriculture showed that ¼ teaspoon to 1 teaspoon of cinnamon with food helps metabolize sugar up to 20 times better.[17] Excess sugar in the blood can lead to fat storage.

Chiles: Add some heat to your food to fire up your metabolism. Capsaicin, the active ingredient in chile peppers, significantly improves fat burning. For more information, consult Tip #13 on page 120.

How to Benefit

It's easy to benefit from the fat-burning ability of spices. Simply start adding more fresh garlic and onions to your vegetable dishes, soups, stir-fries, stews, and curries. Turmeric is excellent in curry dishes. Cinnamon is not only good with sweet foods; it is also excellent in savory dishes and can be added to Asian-inspired foods like curries, stir-fries, and stews. Chiles can be added to almost anything for a blast of heat.

Super Health Bonus

Garlic, onions, and turmeric boost liver function. Turmeric has been shown in study after study to help protect your brain from damage, including diseases like Alzheimer's and Parkinson's. Because cinnamon balances blood sugar levels, it also boosts mood and energy levels. Chile peppers help boost energy as well.

60-Second Weight-Loss Tip #24:
Eat the Top Five Fat-Burning Fruits

Adding more of these surprising fruits to your diet speeds fat loss.

While fruit has many natural healing compounds, sometimes its sugar content can be a problem for people interested in losing weight. However, some fruits actually help you to burn fat. Here are my picks for the Top Five Fat-Burning Fruits.

Avocado: Loaded with healthy omega-9 fatty acids (the same fats found in olive oil, olives, and macadamia nuts), avocados speed the conversion of fat into energy and boost the rate of metabolism.

Coconut: Coconut is rich with medium-chain triglycerides (MCTs), which increase the liver's rate of metabolism by up to 30 percent, according to some experts. They also help keep you full so you're less likely to snack on junk food. As you learned in Tip #19 on page 129, consuming coconut oil aids the functioning of the thyroid gland. Coconut oil, coconut milk (not the low-fat variety), coconut flour, and shredded (unsweetened) coconut all contain MCTs.

Lemons: Excellent liver detoxifiers, lemons also alkalize our body. They may seem acidic based on taste, but in the process of being metabolized by the body, they actually alkalize our bodily fluids and tissues. Maintaining the health of the liver is also imperative to the body's ability to digest and burn fat, since the liver is one of the organs responsible for these functions.

Grapefruit: Many studies confirm that grapefruit is an excellent weight-loss food. In one study at Johns Hopkins University, women who ate grapefruit daily shed almost 20 pounds on average in only 13 weeks, without changing anything else in their diet or lifestyle. Read more about the fat-burning wonders of grapefruit in Tip #31 on page 147.

Tomatoes: Packed with vitamin C and the phytochemical lycopene, tomatoes stimulate the production of the amino acid known as carnitine. In research, carnitine sped up the body's fat-burning capacity by one-third.

How to Benefit

Check out my recipe for Chunky Guacamole on page 254 in the recipe section. I've included many recipes using coconut milk and oil as well. Try my Super Fat-Busting Green Tea Lemonade on page 245. Enjoy a grapefruit for breakfast or as a snack instead of something sweet. Make your own fresh salsa (see recipe on page 255), or add tomatoes to soups, stews, salads, and curries.

Super Health Bonus

Avocado helps prevent heart disease. Coconuts help prevent cancer. Grapefruit gives the liver a boost. Lycopene is a powerful antioxidant that studies show cuts the risk of heart disease by 29 percent.[18]

60-Second Weight-Loss Tip #25:
Eat the Top Five Nuts, Seeds, and Oils

These five nuts, seeds, and oils help your body to burn more fat.

Most people incorrectly assume that eating fat will make them fat. While that may be true of trans fats and hydrogenated fats, there are some excellent food sources of healthy fats that actually help you lose weight. Here are my Top Five Nuts, Seeds, and Oils to burn more fat.

Almonds: Almonds are definitely among the best weight-loss foods. You may recall that women who snacked on 70 almonds daily had a 14 percent waistline reduction, based on research published in the *International Journal of Obesity and Related Metabolic Disorders.*[19] Refer to Tip #15 on page 124 for more information.

Coconut oil: Exciting research by Bruce Fife showed that coconut oil helps to dramatically boost metabolism by resetting the thyroid gland—the body's metabolism gland. Check out Tip #19 on page 129 for more information about this important cooking and baking oil.

Flaxseeds and flaxseed oil: These foods attract oil-soluble toxins that are lodged in the fatty tissues of the body to escort them out.[20]

Olives and olive oil: Being rich in healthy fats, olives and olive oil help to reduce cravings for junk foods and keep you feeling full. In one study, the consumption of olive oil slashed hunger by 70 percent. Research shows that the monounsaturated fats plentiful in olive oil help reduce high blood pressure.[21]

Walnuts: Raw, unsalted walnuts provide your body with essential fatty acids that help burn fat. Walnuts are a rich source of fat-burning omega-3 fatty acids. According to Harvard University research, eating 3 ounces of nuts (like almonds and walnuts) daily helped people lose 1 inch of fat from their waist per month. The scientists at Harvard also found that people who ate 3 ounces of nuts daily were more likely to keep the fat off. Of course, you should avoid salted nuts. Choose raw nuts that are kept refrigerated to prevent the healthy fats they contain from going rancid.

How to Benefit

Snack on raw, unsalted almonds and walnuts throughout the day. Add ground almonds (also called almond meal or almond flour) to your baked goods. Drink almond milk in place of cow's milk. Cook or bake with coconut or olive oil over low to medium heat, not allowing it to smoke. Add flaxseeds and flax oil to smoothies or over cooked vegetable dishes. Don't cook with flax oil. Throw a handful of walnuts on top of your favorite salad.

Super Health Bonus

Eating nuts like almonds and walnuts lowers the risk of a heart attack by 60 percent. Research shows that consuming nuts can be as effective as taking cholesterol-lowering drugs in reducing high cholesterol levels, not to mention that nuts taste better and have no nasty side effects.[22]

60-Second Weight-Loss Tip #26:
Eat Five More Foods That Burn Fat

Add these five foods and beverages to maximize fat loss.

When it comes to burning fat, not all foods are created equal. By now you should be eating more vegetables, cutting out refined sugar, avoiding fast food, and incorporating other dietary changes to lose weight. But there's more you can do to maximize your weight-loss efforts.

Simply adding the following foods to your diet will encourage your body to become a slim and trim fat-burning machine. Proven to help you flush fat, they are an excellent addition to a healthy weight-loss program. Additionally, I've listed the Top Five Fat-Burning Spices, the Top Five Fat-Burning Fruits, and the Top Five Nuts, Seeds, and Oils to Burn More Fat in Tips #23 (page 137), #24 (page 138), and #25 (page 140).

> **Beans and legumes:** Legumes are the best source of fiber of any foods. They help to stabilize blood sugar while keeping you regular. They are also high in potassium, a critical mineral that reduces dehydration and the risk of high blood pressure and stroke. One legume, soy, is particularly good for fat burning. Isoflavones found in soy foods speed

the breakdown of stored fat. In one study, those who consumed high amounts of soy products shed three times more superfluous weight than did their counterparts who ate no soy.[23] But be aware that if you are one of the many people who has an underactive thyroid or is sensitive to soy, it could have the reverse effect, causing you to gain weight instead. Few people have sensitivities to other types of legumes, with the exception of peanuts. Most peanuts are prone to developing aflatoxins—a type of mold that is extremely damaging to health.

Fish and seafood: Fish stimulates the metabolism more than other types of protein-based food. In one study, people who ate fish lost 22 percent more weight than those who ate the same diet but without the fish. Super health bonus: Thanks to the anti-inflammatory omega-3 fatty acids found in fish, you'll reduce your risk of both heart disease and stroke.

Recent research shows that when you eat fish or seafood, you'll stay full for 2 hours longer than you normally would. Fish and seafood increase the body's production of a hormone called leptin that shuts down hunger pangs between meals. Wild salmon is a particularly good fat-burning food because of its high levels of omega-3 fatty acids.

Green tea: Green tea is one of the best fat-fighting superfoods we have. Thanks to a type of catechin called epigallocatechin gallate (EGCG), which has been shown in many studies to increase fat loss, green tea makes the Top Five Foods to Add to Your Diet list. See Tip #17 on page 126 for more information. While it is acid forming, you can offset some of the acidity by adding pH drops or making my recipe for Super Fat-Busting Green Tea Lemonade (see page 245).

Leafy greens: Spinach, spring mix, mustard greens, and other dark leafy greens are good sources of fiber and powerhouses of nutrition. Research demonstrates that their high concentration of vitamins and antioxidants helps prevent hunger while protecting you from heart disease, cancer, cataracts, and memory loss.[24]

How to Benefit

Toss a handful of chickpeas on your salad. Add beans to your soups, stews, curries, and other dishes. I frequently add chickpea flour to my baked goods. Make fish or seafood a regular part of your meals. Ideally, eat them at least three times a week to fully reap their weight-loss benefits. Enjoy 3 or more cups of green tea daily. Eat at least one large leafy green salad daily. Add additional leafy greens to wraps and sandwiches. You can even add a small handful to a smoothie to ramp up its nutritional value. Add kale, collards, or spinach to your soups, stews, curries, or vegetable dishes.

Super Health Bonus

All of these foods have shown tremendous ability to help protect against cancer and heart disease. You can lose weight knowing you're also warding off serious illnesses.

60-Second Weight-Loss Tip #27:
Eat Red, Purple, and Black Foods

The antioxidant anthocyanin causes dramatic weight loss and is found in dark and reddish foods like red or purple grapes, black beans, beets, cherries, and more.

The phytonutrient group called anthocyanins that gives foods their reddish to black appearance also stimulates the burning of stored fat in the body as fuel. A group of laboratory animals fed a high-fat diet along with anthocyanins gained 24 percent less weight than their counterparts fed only the fatty diet, according to research published in *The Journal of Agricultural and Food Chemistry*.[25]

Additional research showed that when obese lab animals were fed a diet rich in blueberries, they lost up to 30 percent more weight around their abdomens than animals fed the same diet minus the blueberries. Steven Bolling, MD, and his researchers published their findings in the *Journal of Medicinal Food*. They believe that anthocyanins, the phytonutrients that give blueberries their blue hue, are responsible for the weight-loss effects.[26]

How to Benefit

Anthocyanins are found in fruits such as dark purple or red grapes, cherries, and berries, including blueberries, blackberries, raspberries, and strawberries. They are also found in black beans and beets.

Super Health Bonus

Not only do anthocyanins help blast fat. Research shows that this potent phytonutrient group also has the capacity to boost short-term memory.[27] So don't be surprised if you're slimmer and have a better memory.

60-Second Weight-Loss Tip #28:
Drink Water with Lemon Juice

Drinking plenty of water with fresh lemon juice helps to flush toxins from fat cells.

There is a beverage that costs only pennies and flushes toxins from fat cells and boosts the liver's ability to metabolize fat. It is not only cheap but is also readily available. What is it? Water with fresh lemon juice.

You may be surprised to learn that the simple addition of fresh lemon juice will help to alkalize your body and boost your fat-burning capacity. It seems contradictory that such an acidic-tasting fruit could alkalize your biochemistry, but it's true.

While lemon tests acidic in a laboratory, it has an alkalizing effect on the body. That's because laboratory tests to determine pH levels don't account for the complex biochemical reactions that occur during digestion. The interaction between a food and our digestive juices, along with mineral and sugar content, determines whether a food has an overall alkalizing or acidifying effect on the body.

To determine whether a food alkalizes or acidifies the body, researchers also look at whether it has an acidic or alkaline ash when burned, since that is essentially what happens to food during metabolism.

Not only does fresh lemon juice help balance your blood chemistry, but its natural phytonutrients also boost liver function by up to 35 percent. And, as you learned earlier, your liver is your body's main fat-metabolizing and detoxifying organ.

How to Benefit

Add the juice of a whole lemon to a large glass of water and drink it first thing in the morning to help your body rehydrate. If it is too tart for you, sweeten it with a few drops of liquid stevia for delicious lemonade. Don't use bottled lemon juice—it is important to use fresh lemon juice only. While it takes only a minute to juice fresh lemons, you can also juice them the night before and store the juice in the refrigerator in a glass jar—absolutely no plastic or metal! Then your lemon juice will be ready for you to add to water and drink when you wake up.

If you don't have access to freshly squeezed lemon juice, you can add 20 pH drops to a large glass of water and drink. Remember to drink at least 1 quart or liter per 50 pounds of body weight (your current weight, not your desired weight). Note that pH drops are sometimes labeled as aerobic oxygen, oxygen, alkaline balance, or sodium chloride drops.

Safety Consideration

After drinking lemon water, swish your mouth out with pure water to prevent the juice from wearing down dental enamel. Alternatively, drink lemon water through a glass or stainless steel straw. Avoid drinking lemon juice if you have an ulcer.

Super Health Bonus

Lemons contain over 20 cancer-fighting compounds, so they will help you lose weight while also reducing your risk of cancer at the same time. That's a serious superfood. You can't get that from bacon.

60-Second Weight-Loss Tip #29:
Get Enough Ellagic Acid

When eaten in moderate amounts, this powerful nutrient found in many fruits, particularly cherries, grapes, and berries, supercharges the liver's ability to break down hormones and toxins and burn fat.

Ellagic acid is a potent phytonutrient that helps stimulate the detoxification systems in the liver to function optimally, thereby helping the liver to eliminate environmental toxins, excess hormones, and food toxins and perform its hundreds of important functions normally.[28]

Its presence in whiskey has caused some people to jokingly claim whiskey as a health food, which, although tempting, is a bit of a stretch. It is far better to obtain ellagic acid from sweet and sour cherries, blueberries, blackberries, chokeberries, strawberries, raspberries, elderberries, black and red currants, and grapes than to ingest alcohol, which is a neurotoxin (meaning it damages brain and nervous system cells) and hormone disruptor. I'm not suggesting that you have to swear off alcohol for life, although people with certain health conditions may benefit from doing so. But alcohol is rich in sugar and strains the liver—both of which defeat weight loss. If your main goal is to slim down, the less alcohol you drink, the better off you'll be.

How to Benefit

Eat sweet and sour cherries, blueberries, blackberries, chokeberries, strawberries, raspberries, elderberries, and black and red currants. Eat grapes in moderate amounts throughout the plan whenever you have a craving for sweets (but not within 3 hours of bedtime). Otherwise, focus on the sour and less sweet fruits more than sweet ones like grapes.

Super Health Bonus

Ellagic acid demonstrates both anticancer and genetic material–protection capabilities. It encourages a healthy rate of apoptosis—the process by which the body seeks out and destroys harmful or damaged cells like cancer cells, helping to reduce the likelihood you'll suffer from cancer.

60-Second Weight-Loss Tip #30:
Eat Cruciferous Vegetables and Leafy Greens

Cruciferous vegetables and leafy greens contain a potent compound that stops your body from storing fat while helping to eliminate toxins.

There is a sulfur compound in cruciferous vegetables that helps to eliminate harmful toxins from your body while signaling your body to stop storing fat. This powerful phytonutrient is called sulforaphane, and research at Nashville's Vanderbilt Medical Center shows that it can increase weight loss by as much as 22 percent.[29] It works by releasing trapped toxins that slow metabolism and increase fat storage within fat cells.

Sulforaphane is found in many foods, including broccoli, cabbage, brussels sprouts, cauliflower, bok choy, and other cruciferous vegetables, as well as dark leafy greens.

Dark leafy greens are also high in one of our favorite minerals—calcium. Kale improves the body's fat detoxification systems by increasing isothiocyanates (ITCs) made from the vegetable's glucosinolates.

How to Benefit

Add more cruciferous vegetables like broccoli, cabbage, brussels sprouts, cauliflower, bok choy, as well as dark leafy greens like kale and collards to your diet. Additionally, garlic and onions also contain sulforaphane.

Safety Suggestion

If you suspect low thyroid function (see Tip #42 on page 177) or have been diagnosed with a low thyroid function, avoid eating cruciferous vegetables raw. However, cooking them destroys the substances that can interfere with thyroid function.

Super Health Bonus

Research shows that collards are among the best foods for lowering cholesterol levels because of their superior ability to bind to bile acids in the intestines. Collards also show excellent anti-cancer properties. Proven to lower the risk of bladder, breast, colon, ovarian, and prostate cancer, kale is among the best superfoods available. So eating more foods rich in sulforaphane will help you balance cholesterol levels and prevent cancer.

60-Second Weight-Loss Tip #31:
Enjoy Grapefruit Daily

When grapefruit is eaten on a daily basis, it can help you to lose up to 20 pounds in 13 weeks.

Grapefruit has long been touted as a superior weight-loss food, but now there's plenty of exciting research to back up the claim. In a study at Johns Hopkins University, women who ate grapefruit daily shed almost 20 pounds in 13 weeks on average. According to researchers, grapefruit contains

12 grams of appetite-suppressing pectin—a special type of fiber found in citrus fruits.[30]

In a 12-week study of 91 overweight adults, eating half a grapefruit daily with or before meals resulted in hunger control and weight loss. People who ate the grapefruit had significantly lower insulin levels (insulin is the fat-hoarding hormone secreted by your pancreas).[31]

Italian research also showed that grapefruit eaten as part of a daily diet boosted metabolic rate enough to burn 12 percent of the daily calories of study participants.[32]

Still further research has shown that a particular phytonutrient group found in grapefruit and other citrus fruits, called terpene limonoids, can benefit weight-loss efforts. There are about 40 types of limonoids alone. Research shows that they significantly improve the liver's ability to eliminate toxins we've inhaled or ingested, including cancer-causing agents.[33]

How to Benefit

Eat one-half to one full grapefruit daily as a snack or about 15 minutes before meals.

Super Health Bonus

Many phytonutrients found in grapefruit, including over 40 limonoids, significantly reduce the risk of cancer, according to research.[34]

60-Second Weight-Loss Tip #32:
Replenish Bowel Flora

Adding critical bacteria to your diet can dramatically boost your weight-loss efforts by restoring bowel health and eliminating infections.

You may be shocked to learn that bacteria are important for weight loss. Before I explain why, I'll share some insights into bacteria and the role they play in your body. Half of the cells in your body are bacterial, the majority of which are beneficial and even essential to the health of your body.

Over 1 trillion bacteria made up of more than 400 different species reside in your intestines. Actually, there are more microorganisms naturally found in your digestive tract than there are cells in your body. An additional 100 trillion microorganisms inhabit our ears, nose, throat, mouth, skin, and other parts of our bodies. This may sound a bit like a scary science fiction movie, but most of these bacteria are necessary to our survival.

Certain types of bacteria, known collectively as probiotics, have a positive impact on your body and its health. They aid digestion and the absorption of essential nutrients, ensure the proper elimination of wastes from the intestines, are involved in the manufacture of important vitamins, control harmful bacteria and yeast populations in the body, and perform other necessary functions.

Adding foods full of bacteria to your diet might not sound appetizing or helpful for weight loss, but if they contain the right types of bacteria, they will dramatically increase fat loss.

Research shows that the ratio of harmful microbes to healthy ones in our gut can influence our weight in a variety of ways, including by:

- Providing us with energy through the breakdown of undigestible carbohydrates in our diet

- Affecting the cellular energy levels of liver and muscle cells

- Affecting the accumulation of fat in our tissue

Thus, it is not surprising that in several studies the gastrointestinal flora of overweight and obese people has been found to differ from that of lean people. And, you've probably guessed it: Overweight and obese individuals tend to have a higher ratio of harmful microbes to beneficial ones.[35]

Research in the journal *Internal and Emergency Medicine* indicates that probiotics may help balance the intestinal bacterial flora in humans, with promising preliminary results in the prevention and treatment of obesity and metabolic disorders.[36]

Many different types of beneficial bacteria may be helpful with weight-loss efforts. One type is known as *Lactobacillus kimchii*. If you're familiar with Korean foods, you may have guessed where you can find this type of bacteria. That's right, it's found in the popular Korean dish kimchi.

How can you tell if you have insufficient probiotic bacteria in your body? Well, there may be no symptoms at all, but more often than not, you'll experience some signs, such as:

- Acne

- Bloating

- Bruising easily

- Cold sores, canker sores, or herpes simplex
- Constipation
- Diarrhea
- Eczema or psoriasis
- Heart disease
- Hemorrhoids
- High cholesterol
- Indigestion
- Intestinal gas
- Irritable bowel syndrome
- Nosebleeds
- Urinary tract infections (also bladder or kidney infections, called cystitis)
- Yeast infections or candida overgrowth

Of course, these conditions and symptoms can be the result of other issues in your body, so you should consult a doctor if you're experiencing any of them. However, the beneficial effects of eating more foods containing naturally present bacteria and/or taking probiotic supplements will often help alleviate many unexpected symptoms. There are no harmful effects of taking them, so they're worth a try.

How to Benefit

Take a probiotic supplement first thing in the morning with your green drink or pH-balanced water, or before bed. Either way, be sure to take it on an empty stomach for the best results. Ideally, choose one that contains *Lactobacillus acidophilus, L. bifidus, Bacillus subtilis, L. casei, L. bulgaris, L. lactis, L. F19, L. rhamnosus, L. plantarum, L. paracasei, L. salivarius, Bifidobacterium bifidum, B. longum,* and *B. infantis.* While you can obtain some probiotics from yogurt, the dairy is acid forming, and most commercial yogurt does not contain live probiotics—even if the label claims otherwise.

Additionally, add fermented foods like kimchi, sauerkraut (be sure it's the real deal since most sauerkraut sold in grocery stores is either not fermented, or the beneficial bacteria are killed during the bottling process), miso, and other naturally fermented foods. Fermented foods are Wise Acid foods that play an important role in your health, so keep them in the maximum 30 percent component of your diet.

Super Health Bonus

Research shows that many types of beneficial bacteria are also involved in maintaining a healthy brain. So while you're repopulating your intestines with friendly bacteria to lose weight, your brain will be getting a boost too.

60-Second Weight-Loss Tip #33:
Add Sprouts to Your Meals

Sprouts significantly boost fat loss and rev up your energy—with almost no calories.

As you learned in Chapter 2, sprouts are nutritional powerhouses. They are loaded with fat-digesting enzymes (and others), vitamins, minerals, protein, and fiber. Plus they contain almost no calories. If you need a reminder about the many excellent reasons to add sprouts to your diet, you can review them in Chapter 2. Many different types of sprouts—including alfalfa, clover, mung bean, radish, broccoli, garlic, and onion—are available in most health food stores or grocery stores. Be sure to wash them before using.

You may be surprised to learn that ancient Aztecs soaked seeds and nuts in water overnight, drained them, then dried them in the sun. While they may not have had the advanced technologies to identify enzymes contained in these foods, they obviously instinctively recognized the power of enzymes. This simple soaking technique not only breaks down natural phytic acid enzyme inhibitors that can irritate the digestive tract, it also activates the fat-burning and digestion-enhancing enzymes found in these foods.

Even if you don't have time to sprout, soak your nuts and seeds overnight in water to maximize their nutritional potential and digestibility. Most nuts will not sprout, but you'll still obtain the benefits of soaking them. I usually soak almonds in water before bed and then drain them in the morning to take with me as a snack during the day. Check out Tip #15 on page 124 to learn more about the fat-reducing benefits of almonds.

How to Benefit

I encourage you to grow your own sprouts. Not only is sprouting really easy, but sprouts are also the ultimate locally grown food. In other words, you'll be doing great things for your body and helping the environment too. Growing your own sprouts is a great way to have a supply of gourmet varieties, to ensure access to high-quality fresh foods year round if you live in a colder climate, and to readily increase the alkalizing and nutritional quality of your diet.

Even if you choose not to grow your own sprouts, you can still obtain their weight-loss benefits by adding them to your daily diet. A handful of alfalfa sprouts on a sandwich or mashed into some guacamole is delicious. Or toss some kelp noodles with a large handful of mung bean sprouts and some grated ginger and tamari (an alternative to soy sauce).

There are many different approaches to sprouting. I prefer the simple jar method using wide-mouthed mason jars. If you opt to grow your own sprouts, you'll need only a few basic supplies to get started. They include:

- Organic sprouting seeds, nuts, legumes, or grains
- Measuring spoons or cups
- Large wide-mouthed jars
- Sprouting lids for jars (They are typically available in most health food stores, and I've also included them on my Web site, www.DrMichelleCook.com, in case you have trouble finding them. Alternatively, you can use cheesecloth and rubber bands over the top of the jars.)

Once you have these items, you're ready to start growing sprouts. You'll soon discover it is absolutely simple.

STEP-BY-STEP INSTRUCTIONS

Step 1: Wash your hands thoroughly before handling seeds of any kind. (This includes seeds, nuts, legumes, and grains. For simplicity I'll be referring to all of these items as "seeds" in the following steps.)

Step 2: Remove any broken or discolored seeds, stones, twigs, or hulls that may have found their way into your sprouting seeds.

Step 3: Place the seeds in the jar—only one type of seed per jar since they grow at different rates, unless you're using special sprouting seed combinations. Follow the amounts specified in the chart on page 154. Use no more than a teaspoon of most seeds or ⅓ cup of beans, since they will absorb water and grow substantially in size. Also, be sure you're using medium to large jars.

Step 4: Cover the seeds with pure water. If you are using a few tablespoons of seeds, cover with at least 1 cup of water. If you are using beans, nuts, or grains, use at least three times as much water: for example, 1 cup of water for $\frac{1}{3}$ cup of mung beans.

Step 5: Let soak for 6 to 12 hours. Often I'll start the soaking them just before going to bed or first thing in the morning.

Step 6: Cover the jar with the sprouting lid or cheesecloth. If you're using cheesecloth, secure it over the top of the jar with a rubber band. Drain off the water.

Step 7: Rinse thoroughly with fresh water and drain off the water again. Set upside down in a clean, cool spot in your kitchen, preferably on a slight angle to allow excess water to drain off.

Step 8: Rinse the sprouts a few times a day. Be sure to drain them well each time.

Step 9 (optional): Once the sprouts are ready to be harvested, place them in a large bowl of cool water and stir them around to loosen hulls and skins from the seeds. They'll usually come to the top so you can remove them. Don't worry about removing every last one. This step helps prevent spoilage and encourages the sprouts to last longer. Drain sprouts well and store them in the refrigerator for a week to 10 days, depending on the sprout type.

TIP: To increase the mineral content of your sprouts, add a piece of kelp or other type of seaweed to the water while the seeds are soaking.

On rare occasions, a batch of seeds won't sprout. Here are some reasons why.

1. The seeds may be too old.
2. The seeds may have been irradiated to destroy bacteria before arriving on grocery or health food store shelves.
3. The seeds may have been exposed to moisture during storage, either at your home or where they were warehoused or sold.
4. The seeds may have been exposed to excessive heat during storage, either at the distribution center, retail outlet, or your home. Foods like oat groats and almonds are often heated in an effort to extend shelf life. This is true of many so-called raw almonds, so be sure you buy your raw almonds from a reputable source.

(continued on page 158)

Simple Sprouting

Seed Type	Amount	Soaking Time	Sprouting Time
Adzuki bean	½ cup	12 hours	3–5 days
Alfalfa seed	3 Tbsp	5 hours	3–6 days
Almond	1½ cups	8–10 hours	1–2 days
Amaranth grain	1 cup	3–5 hours	2–3 days
Broccoli seed	2 Tbsp	8 hours	3–4 days
Buckwheat (hulled)	1 cup	6 hours	1–2 days
Cabbage seed	1 Tbsp	4–6 hours	4–5 days
Chickpeas	1 cup	12–48 hours	2–4 days
Clover seed	3 Tbsp	5 hours	4–6 days
Fenugreek seed	4 Tbsp	6 hours	2–5 days
Kale seed	4 Tbsp	4–6 hours	4–6 days
Kamut grain	1 cup	12 hours	2 days

Approximate Yield	Sprout Length at Harvest	More Information
4 cups	½"–1½"	Best if rinsed a few times a day.
3–4 cups	1"–2"	To "green" the leaves, place in indirect sunlight on last day of sprouting.
2 cups	Up to ⅛"	Most often eaten just soaked.
3 cups	Up to ¼"	Best if rinsed a few times a day.
2 cups	1"–2"	Rinse a few times a day. Place in indirect sunlight on last day of sprouting.
2 cups	⅓"–½"	Best if rinsed every 30 minutes for the first few hours. Soak for no longer than 6 hours.
1½ cups	1"–2"	Rinse 2 to 3 times a day, shaking vigorously.
3–3½ cups	½"–1"	To make them easier to digest, soak longer. Rinse often during sprouting process.
3–4 cups	1"–2"	"Green" leaves in indirect sunlight on last day.
2½–3 cups	1"	Bitter if left to grow past 1".
3–4 cups	¾"–1"	Rinse 2 to 3 times a day.
2–3 cups	¼"–½"	Rinse often. Can be used to make sprouted bread.

Seed Type	Amount	Soaking Time	Sprouting Time
Lentil	¾ cup	8 hours	2–3 days
Mustard seed	3 Tbsp	5 hours	3–5 days
Oats (whole, hulled grain)	1 cup	8 hours	1–2 days
Onion seed	1 Tbsp	4–6 hours	4–5 days
Pinto bean	1 cup	12 hours	3–4 days
Pumpkin seed	1 cup	6 hours	1–2 days
Quinoa grain	1 cup	3–4 hours	2–3 days
Radish seed	3 Tbsp	6 hours	3–5 days
Rye grain	1 cup	6–8 hours	2–3 days
Sesame seed (hulled)	1 cup	8 hours	Less than 1 day
Spelt grain	1 cup	6 hours	1–2 days
Sunflower, hulled	1 cup	6–8 hours	Less than 1 day
Teff seed	1 cup	3–4 hours	1–2 days
Wheat grain	1 cup	8–10 hours	2–3 days

Approximate Yield	Sprout Length at Harvest	More Information
3–4 cups	½"– 1"	Rinse often. Be sure to remove broken or split lentils prior to soaking.
3 cups	½"–1½"	"Green" in indirect sun on last day of sprouting.
1 cup	Up to ⅛"	Rinse 3 times a day. Be sure to use whole, hulled grain that has not been steamed. Can be difficult to sprout.
1½–2 cups	1"–2"	Rinse a few times a day.
3–4 cups	½"–1"	Rinse a few times a day minimum.
1½–2 cups	Up to ⅛"	It's fine to use them after soaking only. May not sprout.
3 cups	Up to ½"	Rinse thoroughly prior to soaking for best taste.
3–4 cups	¾"–2"	Rinse thoroughly prior to soaking for best taste.
3 cups	½"–¾"	Rinse a few times a day. Don't leave in overly warm environment.
2 cups	n/a	Will not sprout, but soaking increases nutrients and digestibility.
2 cups	Up to ¼"	Replaces wheat in recipes.
2 cups	¼"–½"	Skim off skins after soaking.
2½–3 cups	Up to ⅛"	Teff can be hard to sprout because of the seed's tiny size, which can escape even the finest mesh sprouting lid. Try cheesecloth held in place by an elastic band over a glass jar.
2–3 cups	¼"–¾"	Use to make sprouted grain breads.

5. Many refined grains like oats, pearl barley, rice, and debittered quinoa will not sprout because of the refining process.

6. The seeds may need additional or less soaking time. Refer to the sprouting chart on page 154.

7. Insects may have damaged the seeds.

60-Second Weight-Loss Tip #34:
Add the Ancient Grain Quinoa to Your Diet

Quinoa is a fat-busting superfood that helps you balance blood sugar and lose weight.

A staple of the ancient Incas, who revered it as sacred, quinoa (pronounced KEEN-wah) is not a true grain but a seed. Surprisingly, it is related to spinach and Swiss chard. If you're not already enjoying this delicious food, there are many reasons to start.

Unlike most grains that contribute to weight gain and are incomplete proteins (they lack one or more of the essential amino acids that make up a complete protein), quinoa is a complete protein. Quinoa packs an amino acid punch while still being alkalizing, making it a great weight- loss food. It is rich in nutrients, including manganese, iron, magnesium, B vitamins, and fiber—all of which are needed to burn fat.

In studies, quinoa is a proven aid for migraine sufferers, likely because of its magnesium and riboflavin content. Magnesium helps relax muscles and riboflavin helps reduce the frequency of migraine attacks and improves energy metabolism within brain and muscle cells. Fewer migraines and muscle healing help ensure you can stick to your exercise program and feel better. Like its grain counterparts, quinoa lessens the risk for heart disease and helps with heart arrhythmias.

It contains the building blocks for superoxide dismutase—an important antioxidant that protects the energy centers of your cells from free radical damage. Stronger cell energy centers means less fatigue for you and more energy to burn fat.

It cooks in under 20 minutes, making it a much healthier alternative to white rice and much faster to prepare than most whole grains. Plus, it is gluten free, which makes it good for anyone suffering from celiac or autoimmune disorders. It's also a good source of the amino acid trypto-phan—you know, the one that helps with melatonin production, which helps improve sleep quality. Additionally, it is high in lysine, which helps with tissue repair and growth. It also helps ward off cold sores.

Quinoa is rich in fiber, which helps eliminate harmful toxins from your bowels before they can be resorbed, helps with fat loss, and protects against gallstones, according to the *American Journal of Gastroenterology.*[37]

How to Benefit

Quinoa is versatile. Add coconut or almond milk to cooked quinoa for a delicious hot breakfast "cereal." Add cooked vegetables like onions, red bell peppers, and squash with a few herbs for a delicious meatless meal. Or add finely chopped onion, cucumber, green bell peppers, and toma-toes with some oregano and lemon juice for a delicious and satisfying take on Greek salad.

I've included instructions for cooking Basic Quinoa on page 290 of this book. Additionally, I've included many other delicious breakfast, lunch, and dinner recipes for quinoa in Part 3.

Super Health Bonus

Quinoa's protein and superoxide dismutase contents make it a high-energy food. It will boost your cells' energy centers, which translates into more energy for you in addition to more energy for fat burning. What's more, quinoa may even help reduce the risk of type 2 diabetes, thanks to its magnesium stores. Magnesium helps activate more than 500 enzymes in your body, including those involved in insulin secretion and the body's use of sugar.

60-Second SUCCESS STORY

Kate Acton

Age: **29**
Location: **Boston**
Occupation: **Nanny**

Total Weight Lost:
10 pounds

Total Inches Lost:
18.75

"My clothes fit so much better."

How I Got Here:

Kate shared: "Before I started the program, I was feeling tired and bloated, and I had low self-esteem. I was irritable and had aches and pains in my knees, hips, and legs. I had digestive complaints including gas, bloating, nausea, and constipation. I was breaking out and having minor seasonal allergies. I felt way older than my age." Having studied nutrition and microscopy, Kate already knew some of the issues with her diet and lifestyle. "I, like most Americans," she says, "was addicted to sugar and caffeine. I woke up in the morning craving sugar and went to bed with a stomachache from consuming too many sugars. I felt bloated, and you could see it in my face. I would be too tired to exercise and more often opt for a nap over exercise. I needed coffee every day."

She was highly motivated to try 60 Seconds to Slim because it was a new spin on a type of program she had tried before: "I had success before by restoring my pH balance but had fallen off the wagon and truly forgot how it felt to be energized and healthy. I let my old food addictions take over, and it wasn't until I was in pain and desperate to lose weight for my wedding that I realized this is not how I wanted to start my life with my future husband. I wanted to be a beautiful, alkaline bride on my wedding day.

"My goal was to lose the acidic fat I had built up over the past few years. I wanted clear skin, a clear mind, and an abundance of energy. I wanted to create healthy blood and a healthy body for my future as a wife and eventually, a mother."

Progress Report:

Because eating an alkaline diet was familiar to Kate, she knew what to expect. "The first few days were tough because I felt hungry even though I knew I was getting enough good fats and greens. I was drinking my ionized water and greens and I had some detox symptoms such as a headache.

My energy was really low at the start of the program. I would get over 8 hours of sleep and still feel tired when I woke up. I needed caffeine to get through the day and would often take naps. After the first week I began to have more energy. The fog that I seemed to constantly be in lifted and the aches and pains went away. My bloating went away and my bowel movements were regular and green! *[Michelle's note: This is usually a sign that the liver and gallbladder are cleansing.]* My overall sense of well-being and self-esteem improved greatly. My skin continues to improve and my clothes fit so much better. I am falling asleep earlier and getting up earlier. I don't feel the need for a nap in the middle of the day, and I have more energy than I ever got from coffee. I am excited to continue my journey of alkalizing and balancing my body. I know this will help me spiritually and physically."

(continued)

Beyond:

"Besides the weight loss and increase in energy, I am relieved of pain! This is really big for me since I don't think I realized how much pain I was in until it was gone. No wonder I was irritable. I am looking forward to being able to run and work out without pain. Come to think of it, I am happy I can live each day without any aches and pain. Good-bye, inflammation."

In addition to reducing inflammation, Kate shared that her mood received a tremendous boost: "I was very irritable before the program. I was also more introverted since I didn't like how I felt or looked. Now, just 1 month later, I am smiling more, finding happiness in the little things,

and just feel more relaxed. I am definitely able to experience more joy.

"It has been a long time since I have been able to lose 10 pounds and keep them off. I do need to lose more, but I am so motivated to continue these lifestyle changes that I am excited about it instead of dreading the 'work,' as I used to do. If I continue to alkalize, my body will balance itself and I will find my ideal weight."

Kate is still following the 60 Seconds to Slim program and has made it a way of life. She adds: "I do need to continue to increase my workouts. Other than that, I need to remember a phrase I've heard many times: 'Nothing tastes as good as good health feels.'"

Chapter 5

Week 3: STRATEGIZE

Adopt These Tips and Tricks to Boost Weight Loss

During Week 3, you will learn about the best timing tricks and fat-burning strategies to help you maximize the amount of weight you'll lose. You'll discover the best ways to supercharge your body's pH-balancing abilities, balance hormone mechanisms, power up digestion, and improve your body's detoxification pathways that burn fat. Choose all or at least five of these strategies this week and gradually work them into your new, healthier lifestyle.

Here are the 60-Seconds Weight-Loss Tips you will learn this week:

35. Drink Diluted Cranberry Juice (page 166)

This little-known detox trick quickly and effectively melts fat and targets cellulite.

36. Eat Small Meals Frequently (page 168)

Eating frequently throughout the day is a simple food-timing trick that sends messages to your brain to release fat stores.

37. Eat Carbs Before 3 p.m. (page 169)

Eating carbs before 3 p.m. enables you to enjoy them periodically without worrying about their effects on your belly, thighs, and hips.

38. Jump-Start Weight Loss with Interval Training (page 170)

Varying your exercise routine to include interval training ramps up fat loss by 400 percent.

39. Drink Nothing but Water for 40 Minutes after Exercise (page 172)

Sticking to water for 40 minutes after exercise boosts fat burning.

40. Get More Sleep (page 173)

Get at least 7 hours a night to burn more fat.

41. Add Lymph-Cleansing Strategies (page 175)

Remove excess fat and cellulite with these clarifying techniques.

42. Top Thyroid-Boosting Strategies (page 177)

Reset your thyroid gland and bolster your metabolism with these methods.

43. Listen to Your Body's Hunger Signals (page 179)

Low-calorie dieting and skipping meals actually make you fatter.

44. Eliminate the Microbe That May Be Making You Fat (page 180)

Eliminating the yeast Candida albicans *helps your body shed weight.*

45. Practice Mindful Eating (page 184)

Eating more slowly and being attentive to what you consume help you feel full on less food.

46. Head Out for a Walk (page 185)

Walk daily and you can lose 25 pounds in a year—without changing anything else.

47. Add Resistance Training (page 186)

Resistance training, like weight lifting, results in a 73 percent increase in fat burning for hours afterward.

48. Visualize Yourself Thin (page 187)

Think yourself thin by taking a few moments to visualize what you'll look like when you reach your desired weight.

49. Address Emotional Issues (page 189)

Learn how to release your pent-up negative emotions linked with excess weight.

50. Support Your Stress Glands (page 191)

The following techniques reverse damage to the stress glands and balance the hormones that cause weight gain.

51. Adopt Liver-Boosting Strategies (page 195)

Heal fatty liver disease, an underlying health condition that could be making you fat.

52. Eat Breakfast (page 202)

Eighty percent of overweight people skip breakfast. Eat breakfast and dramatically improve weight loss.

53. Breathe Deeply to Halt Fat-Gaining Hormones (page 203)

Breathing deeply reduces stress hormones linked to weight gain in seconds.

60-Second Weight-Loss Tip #35:
Drink Diluted Cranberry Juice

This little-known detox trick quickly and effectively melts fat and targets cellulite.

This trick hones in on your lymphatic system. Before we explore this valuable weight-loss strategy, let's first explore the lymphatic system.

The lymphatic system is a network that includes fluid-filled tubes, glands, lymph nodes, the spleen, thymus gland, and tonsils. This system bathes our cells and carries the body's cellular sewage away from the tissues and moves it into the blood where it can be filtered by the liver and kidneys. This sewage is made up of any number of things, including the normal by-products of our daily bodily processes, drugs, pollutants, food additives, pesticides, and other toxins that we inhale or ingest.

There is three times more lymph fluid in our bodies than there is blood. But, unlike the blood, which has the heart to pump it throughout the body, the lymph system relies on deep breathing and exercise.

A recent study found that 80 percent of overweight women have sluggish lymphatic systems and that getting these systems flowing smoothly is the key to easy weight loss and improved feelings of well-being.[1]

If we breathe shallowly (most people do), don't get sufficient movement, or are exposed to the many pollutants in our air, food, and water, our lymph system can become sluggish.

This sluggishness causes fluid to back up, resulting in bloated tissue that contains excessive amounts of toxins. Many health experts also link this fluid backup with the formation of cellulite since the fluid "sticks" to fat cells. Additionally, bloated cells and tissues prevent the proper cellular absorption of nutrients and oxygen, which starves them. When your cells are starved of oxygen and nutrients, your body triggers feelings of hunger and cravings that cause you to eat more. We may eat more food in an effort to satisfy our cravings, but rarely do we eat the nutrient-dense foods are bodies are crying out for.

One of the best foods to get a sluggish lymphatic system moving is cranberry juice—not the sugar-laden variety found in most grocery stores, though. Choose pure, unsweetened cranberry juice. It is loaded with beneficial phytonutrients like flavonoids, malic acid, citric acid, and quinic acid.

Based on the research of naturopath Ann Louise Gittleman, cranberry juice emulsifies stubborn fat deposits in the lymphatic system so they can be broken down and removed from the body.

When cranberry juice is made with fresh, unheated cranberries, it also contains many natural enzymes that also help break down fat deposits.

LYMPH QUIZ

How do you know if your lymphatic system might be playing a role in your weight? There are many signs of an overburdened lymphatic system. Take the following quiz to help you decide if your lymph system needs support.

Are you overweight? _____

Do you have cellulite or fatty deposits? _____

Do you suffer from aches and pains? _____

Have you been diagnosed with fibromyalgia, chronic fatigue syndrome, multiple sclerosis, lupus, or another chronic immune system disorder? _____

Have you ever yo-yo dieted? _____

Do you feel bloated or do areas of your body seem bloated or pudgy? _____

Are you prone to lumps or growths on your body? _____

Do you experience abdominal bloating? _____

Do you experience eye puffiness? _____

If you answered yes to one or more of the above questions, your lymphatic system may benefit from a tune-up.

How to Benefit

Add unsweetened and diluted cranberry juice to your diet and drink it throughout the day. Most cranberry "juice" sold in grocery stores is actually a cranberry cocktail loaded with sugar and contains almost no cranberries. Instead, opt for a 100 percent pure cranberry juice. Dilute 1 part cranberry juice with about 4 or 5 parts water. So, for example, start with ½ cup of cranberry juice and add 2 cups of water. It has a tart taste, but your tastebuds will adapt over time. Alternatively, you can throw a handful or two of fresh or frozen cranberries into the blender with some water and blend.

Learn other lymph-boosting foods and strategies in Tip #41 on page 175.

Super Health Bonus

Cranberry juice contains the phytonutrient malic acid, which helps to counteract pain, particularly in people suffering from fibromyalgia. Many of my clients have had dramatic reductions in or a complete reversal of their fibromyalgia symptoms when they address their sluggish lymphatic system.

60-Second Weight-Loss Tip #36:
Eat Small Meals Frequently

Eating frequently throughout the day is a simple food-timing trick that sends messages to your brain to release fat stores.

Did you know that timing your food is the key to telling your brain to release fat? It's true. Eating small amounts frequently throughout the day, such as three meals and two snacks between meals, actually prevents your body from making the hormone ghrelin. Without ghrelin you feel full and your body starts to release its fat stores.

Ghrelin is a hormone called a peptide that is primarily secreted by the stomach (it's also secreted by the pancreas and the pituitary gland in the brain). It sends messages to your brain telling you that you are hungry in order to stimulate appetite. Ghrelin levels tend to increase before meals and decrease after eating.

When you eat small amounts throughout the day in the form of three smaller meals and snacks between meals, ghrelin is reduced or not secreted at all, thereby reducing hunger and cravings.

In some bariatric procedures performed for weight loss, ghrelin levels are reduced, but it isn't necessary to go through invasive surgery to tame your hunger hormone.

How to Benefit

All you need to do to benefit from this food-timing trick is to eat small amounts frequently throughout the day. If you haven't eaten anything for 2 hours, you need to eat again. Ideally, combine some protein and nonstarchy vegetables to obtain the best results. (Good proteins to snack on include nuts, seeds, tofu, avocado, sprouts, fish, or poultry.) If your schedule is busy (and whose isn't these days?), then you'll benefit from preparing some snacks in advance so they are ready to eat between meals. You can soak raw, unsalted almonds overnight, drain them in the morning, and take them to go. Celery sticks with almond butter and a few unsulphured raisins can be prepared ahead of time. You can find unsulphured raisins at your local health food store. Apple slices with avocado or almond butter are another excellent choice. (Hint: If you're slicing the apple ahead of time, drizzle a little lemon juice on it to prevent browning.) For a great, portable, savory snack, try black beans tossed with a little minced onion, chopped celery, lemon juice, and a dash of sea salt.

Super Health Bonus

By following this simple food-timing trick, you'll also experience more energy and balanced moods throughout the day. Your energy levels are closely linked to blood sugar levels. Eat frequently throughout the day and you'll automatically balance blood sugar levels and feel your energy soar.

60-Second Weight-Loss Tip #37:
Eat Carbs before 3 p.m.

Eating carbs before 3 p.m. enables you to enjoy them periodically without worrying about their effects on your belly, thighs, and hips.

Eating lots of sugars and starches is a definite recipe for weight gain, but you can eat the healthier carbs like fruit and whole grains without gaining weight or interfering with your weight-loss efforts if you know the best time of day to eat them. Research shows that eating any starchy carbs earlier in the day, before 3 p.m. to be exact, will boost your energy and won't add fat to your body.[2]

Eat nonstarchy vegetables as your carbs of choice after 3 p.m. to help maintain your weight-loss efforts.

How to Benefit

It's still best to avoid sweets and white starchy foods like pasta, white rice, and white potatoes at all times of day. Focus on whole grains like quinoa, spelt, kamut, buckwheat, or brown rice. But if you must eat something sweet or one of the white starchy foods, be sure you eat it in the morning or early afternoon, before 3 p.m. That said, you should still aim to eat the healthier grain options you have been adding to your plate on this plan before 3 p.m. as well. That will help get even the most stubborn fat to budge. After 3 p.m., focus on protein and veggies—leafy greens, cruciferous vegetables, tomatoes, bell peppers—almost any vegetable that isn't starchy, like potatoes. You can also choose fruit that is low in sugar and carbohydrates, such as berries. Remember that when you are trying to lose weight, moderation is still important no matter what you are eating.

Super Health Bonus

Although I recommend limiting when in the day you consume carbs, be sure you don't cut them out of your diet entirely. By continuing to eat some healthy grains and seeds (quinoa is actually a seed), you'll give your body the components it needs to make healthy neurotransmitters—the brain hormones that help you to maintain balanced moods and to feel great. That's why so many people feel anxious, depressed, or irritable on low-carb programs. Their brains don't have the building blocks for hormones like serotonin, the "feel-good" hormone. By eating healthy carbs you'll balance your moods and feel less anxious. Just be smart about what time of day you eat them in order to maximize weight loss.

60-Second Weight-Loss Tip #38:
Jump-Start Weight Loss with Interval Training

Varying your exercise routine to include interval training ramps up fat loss by 400 percent.

Brisk walking is a great exercise to help build muscle and cardiovascular health, but did you know that you can boost your fat-burning ability just by tweaking your walking routine a bit? Interval walking is a simple way of boosting your fat-burning abilities. You simply walk for brief bursts at a high-intensity pace, then slow down to a more manageable pace, and repeat with brief bursts at the high-intensity pace again. Research shows that interval walking burns three times more fat than nonstop high-intensity exercise.[3] That means you get results faster without having to work as long or as hard.

There's still another option that will help you get an even bigger fat burn for your efforts: Add hills to your outdoor workout or an incline option on your treadmill. You'll use different muscles, increasing the ability of more muscles to burn fat, and you'll also be doing a type of interval walking—regular walking interspersed with hills that add intensity to your workout.

How to Benefit

Lace up your walking shoes! It's easy to implement this tip. Choose the option that feels best for you. If you live in a flat area and plan to walk outdoors, well, interval walking with bursts of faster and slower walking will obviously be the choices for you. If you prefer to walk indoors on a treadmill, mix things up with periodic "hills" or "inclines" on your treadmill.

Time	Activity	Intensity
0:00–5:00	Warmup (5 minutes)	Keep an easy pace, as in a leisurely stroll.
5:00–6:00	Moderate walking (1 minute)	You are breathing harder but can still talk in complete sentences.
6:00–6:30	Fast walking (30 seconds)	Walk as if you are late for an appointment. You may feel breathless but should be able to manage short yes/no responses.
Alternate between 1 minute of moderate walking and 30 seconds of fast walking 13 times, or for 19 minutes and 30 seconds.		
25:30–30:00	Cooldown (4½ minutes)	Keep an easy pace, as in a leisurely stroll.

Doing what fits best with your personality is the best way to ensure you stick with interval training.

It's hard to recommend a one-size-fits-all fitness program since your fitness level will depend on how active or sedentary you were before starting the 60 Seconds to Slim program; however, great places to look for interval-training workouts are the Web sites of popular fitness magazines, such as Prevention.com. Just remember that interval walking can exert you more than your regular routine, so be sure to start at a speed and workout duration that are going to push you a little, but not allow you to overdo it. If you can comfortably walk at a steady pace for 20 minutes or more, this basic interval walk may be a great place for you to start. All you'll need is a watch and a pair of sneakers.

Do this walk two or three times per week, with regular steady-paced cardio on the other days of the week. As you get stronger, you can up the intensity of the intervals or walk for longer to continue challenging yourself. This schedule is also compatible with strength training twice per week. See Tip #47 on page 186 for a fat-incinerating timing trick that brings your cardio and strength routines together.

Super Health Bonus

In addition to building muscle and losing fat, you'll improve your heart health by improving cardiovascular strength and stamina.

60-Second Weight-Loss Tip #39:
Drink Nothing but Water for 40 Minutes after Exercise

Imbibing only water for 40 minutes after exercise boosts fat burning.

When you eat after working out is a factor that plays a major role in whether you'll lose weight—and also how much. So knowing the ideal time to eat after your workouts is essential knowledge if you want to blast the pounds.

Studies at the Netherlands Institute for Brain Research, among others, show that eating or drinking anything other than water within 40 minutes of working out will work against your best weight-loss efforts. The scientists found that keeping adrenaline-rich blood in your trouble spots revs up the fat-burning effects of the enzyme lipase by as much as 51 percent. Eating or drinking anything other than water during those critical 40 minutes actually moves blood to your digestive system and away from fatty areas, negating your best exercise and nutrition efforts.

How to Benefit

To keep lipase-carrying blood circulating in your muscles and not your digestive tract, drink plenty of alkaline water after exercising, particularly after exercise that focuses on your trouble spots like your belly, butt, or thighs. Skip the sports drinks to drop the pounds. Don't eat or drink any-thing other than water for at least 40 minutes after exercising. Knowing the ideal time to eat and drink after working out can really maximize your fat-busting efforts! It works whether you go for a brisk walk or lift some canned goods—you know, the ones you're no longer eating that now serve as excellent weights.

Super Health Bonus

Not only will you reap the best rewards of your exercise, but you'll also help to alkalize your body further by drinking alkaline water during this time. I've heard many people complain that they can't find the time to fit in all the alkaline water they know they should be drinking, but this strategy gives your rehydration efforts a serious boost.

60-Second Weight-Loss Tip #40:
Get More Sleep

Get at least 7 hours a night to burn more fat.

It's true: You can sleep your way slim. Research shows that people who are sleep deprived are more likely to experience intense sugar cravings, the inability to feel full after eating plentiful amounts of food, compulsive overeating, lean muscle loss, impaired ability to burn carbo-hydrates, and a decrease in physical activity.[4] Those six things are huge barriers to weight loss, so if you're not getting enough sleep, you could be thwarting all your best efforts to eat healthy and exercise. Fatigue caused from sleep deprivation slows your metabolism—your body's means of burning fat.[5]

Additional research at the University of Chicago found that well-rested women had faster metabolic rates and ate 15 percent less food each day than those who didn't get a good night's sleep.[6]

Significant amounts of research show that we need at least 7 to 8 hours of sleep each night, although some people need more than that. And if you're nurturing a sleep debt, then even that amount won't be enough. Impressive research from William C. Dement, MD, PhD, the author of *The Promise of Sleep,* shows that our bodies remember when we don't get enough sleep and keep track until we make up the amount. It's like a bank account. If you don't get enough sleep on occasion or on a regular basis, it's like you've made withdrawals from your sleep account. If you don't make up the hours soon afterward, your sleep account goes into negative amounts. So, it's important to prevent a sleep debt by making up lost sleep as soon as possible.[7]

You may already notice that you are sleeping better now that you have a regular exercise routine and are eating healthfully. But what if you just can't get to sleep? Exciting research from neurologist and author of *Life's a Smelling Success* Alan R. Hirsch, MD, found that smelling lavender calmed the entire nervous system in only 1 minute, helping people to feel sleepier.[8]

How to Benefit

Get into a regular evening ritual by dimming lights and limiting exposure to screens in the hour before you plan to sleep. This way, your body will start knowing that it is bedtime and help you to fall asleep. Electronic devices like televisions, smartphones, and laptops emit blue light that can disrupt your sleep cycles if used right before bed. Go to sleep at the same time every night and try to get at least 7 or 8 hours of sleep, waking at the same time each morning. To feel sleepier, spray your pillowcase or sheets with some pure lavender water (preferable to the oil, since lavender essential oil may stain sheets) or place a few drops of oil on a tissue on your end table.

Make sure you're using 100 percent pure lavender essential oil or lavender water or fragrance, not synthetically scented water. These fakes have no beneficial properties and can actually expose you to harmful neurotoxins. Most health food stores sell a natural option made from real lavender.

Super Health Bonus

Getting sufficient sleep not only reduces your weight and hunger, but it also improves your energy, focus, and alertness during the day. This both enhances your performance at work and reduces the risk you'll be involved in a motor vehicle accident, which is closely linked to sleep deprivation.

60-Second Weight-Loss Tip #41:
Add Lymph-Cleansing Strategies

Remove excess fat and cellulite with these clarifying techniques.

If you're following Tip #35 (see page 166), you're already familiar with the lymphatic system. If not, the lymphatic system, or lymph system as it is also called, is made up of glands, lymph nodes, the spleen, thymus gland, and tonsils. It bathes our body's cells and carries the body's cellular sewage away from the tissues to the blood, where it can be filtered by two of the body's main detoxification organs: the liver and the kidneys. This sewage is made up of the by-products of our bodily processes, over-the-counter and prescription drugs, illicit drugs, cigarette toxins, other airborne pollutants, food additives, pesticides, and other toxins.

A recent study found that 80 percent of women have sluggish lymphatic systems and that getting them flowing smoothly is the key to easy weight loss and improved feelings of well-being. Another study found that women with cellulite showed lymphatic system deficiencies.[9]

If you're not sure if your lymphatic system is playing a role in your weight, take the quiz on page 167 to learn about some of the symptoms.

How to Benefit

In addition to following Tip #35 on page 166, if you suspect that a sluggish lymphatic system is playing a role in your weight, there are numerous things you can do to get your lymph flowing smoothly.

1. **Breathe deeply.** Our bodies have three times more lymph fluid than blood, yet no organ to pump it. Your lymph system relies on the

pumping action of deep breathing to help it transport toxins into the blood before they are detoxified by your liver. So breathe in that sweet smell of healing oxygen. Breathe out toxins.

2. **Get moving.** Exercise also ensures the lymph system flows properly. The best kind is rebounding on a mini trampoline, which can dramatically improve lymph flow, but stretching and aerobic exercise also work well.

3. **Drink plenty of water.** Without adequate water, lymph fluid cannot flow properly. To help ensure the water is readily absorbed by your cells, I frequently add some fresh lemon juice or oxygen or pH drops.

4. **Forget the soda, trash the neon-colored sports drinks, and drop the sugar-laden fruit "juices."** These sugar-, color-, and preservative-laden beverages add to the already overburdened workload your lymph system must handle.

5. **Eat more raw fruit on an empty stomach.** The enzymes and acids in fruit are powerful lymph cleansers. Eat them on an empty stomach for best digestion and maximum lymph-cleansing benefits. Most fruits are digested within 30 minutes or so and quickly help you feel better.

6. **Eat plenty of green vegetables.** Greens will help you to get adequate chlorophyll to purify your blood and lymph system.

7. **Eat raw, unsalted nuts and seeds.** These will power up your lymph with adequate fatty acids. Choose from walnuts, almonds, hazelnuts, macadamias, Brazil nuts, flaxseeds, sunflower seeds, and pumpkin seeds.

8. **Drink a few lymph-boosting herbal teas daily.** Astragalus, echinacea, goldenseal, pokeroot, and wild indigo root tea are all good choices. Consult an herbalist or a natural medicine specialist before combining two or more herbs or if you're taking any medications or suffer from any serious health conditions. Avoid using herbs while pregnant or lactating and avoid long-term use of any herb without first consulting a qualified professional.

9. **Brush dry skin before showering.** Use a natural bristle brush. Brush your dry skin in circular motions upward from the feet to the torso and from the fingers to the chest. You want to work in the same direction as your lymph flows—toward the heart.

10. **Alternate hot and cold water in the shower for several minutes.**
    The heat dilates the blood vessels and the cold causes them to
    contract. Avoid this type of therapy if you have a heart or blood
    pressure condition or if you are pregnant.

11. **Get a gentle massage.** Studies show that a gentle massage can push
    up to 78 percent of stagnant lymph back into circulation. Massage
    frees trapped toxins. You can also try a lymph drainage massage.
    It is a special form of massage that specifically targets lymph flow in
    the body. Whatever type of massage you choose, make sure it is
    gentle. Too much pressure may feel good on the muscles, but it
    doesn't have the same lymph-stimulating effects.

Super Health Bonus

There are countless benefits to getting your lymphatic system moving more
efficiently, including more energy, less pain, and improved detoxification.

60-Second Weight-Loss Tip #42:
Top Thyroid-Boosting Strategies

Reset your thyroid gland and bolster your metabolism with these methods.

   Imagine how great it would be to simply reboot your body when it starts
to function less efficiently, enabling it to burn more fat. Here are some simple strategies to help you reset your thyroid gland, the body's main metabolism gland, when it's not operating up to par.

   The thyroid gland is a butterfly-shaped gland located at the base of
your neck, just below the Adam's apple. It is called the metabolism gland
because it secretes hormones that control and are involved in metabolic
activity taking place in every cell of your body. While many people have
heard about underactive thyroid (also called hypothyroidism), they may not
know how it is linked to weight gain. Simply put, a sluggish thyroid leads to
sluggish metabolism, as well as a slow digestive process, which is often impli-
cated in weight gain. The good news is that you can do all kinds of simple,
natural things to give your thyroid a boost. Not only will they help with

weight management, but they may also help you feel more energized, less achy, and even more interested in your daily life and routine. Resetting your thyroid can have all of these benefits and more.

How to Benefit

Food choice is frequently the key to both sluggish and efficient thyroid function. Foods to avoid include the raw form of vegetables in the goitrogen family, such as broccoli, cauliflower, kale, cabbage, brussels sprouts, and soy. Before you get all excited about your new excuse to avoid broccoli and brussels sprouts, know that they are both safe and valuable dietary additions when they are cooked. The cooking process inactivates the goitrogens that negatively affect your thyroid gland. So eat your cooked cauliflower in a delicious dairy-free curry.

You can also add pumpkin seeds, beans, almonds, and cold-water/fatty fish to your diet (see more on this in Tip #26 on page 141) to ensure you are getting enough of the amino acid tyrosine, as well as copper, zinc, and selenium, which are important minerals for healthy thyroid function. Fish is also a good source of healthy essential fatty acids that support thyroid function. These fatty acids can also be found in flaxseeds and walnuts. Look to the sea for iodine-rich sea vegetables (most us know them as seaweed) such as dulse, kelp, and nori. These are often found in Japanese cuisine such as sushi or in dried form at grocery and health food stores. Try to eat a small amount of sea vegetables daily.

Eat more coconut oil (more on this in Tip #19 on page 129). It is a great substitute for butter, margarine, and cooking oils, has far more health benefits, and stimulates the thyroid while lowering cholesterol. Coconut oil is an excellent health-promoting fat that boosts weight loss.

You can also supplement with the natural amino acid carnitine, which can be quite helpful for resetting the thyroid gland. To learn more about this valuable nutrient, see Tip #63 on page 224.

Super Health Bonus

You're already following the 60 Seconds to Slim program, which means you are eating more fiber and drinking more water. Congratulations! By promoting faster elimination of digestive wastes and keeping yourself hydrated, you are also boosting your thyroid function.

60-Second Weight-Loss Tip #43:
Listen to Your Body's Hunger Signals

Low-calorie dieting and skipping meals actually make you fatter.

Those of you who have read my other books know that I am a big fan of enzymes and the important and amazing functions they play in our health, including weight loss. When I refer to enzymes, I am talking about the many enzymes we make in our bodies, as well as enzymes we ingest from food sources, such as vegetables and fruits. They all serve different purposes.

Consider the enzyme lipoprotein lipase (LPL), which is produced by the body. The purpose of LPL is to gather fat found in our blood and store it in fat cells. Science has shown that LPL levels are determined in part by heredity and that children of obese parents have higher levels of LPL and are therefore more likely to store fat. Interestingly, the harder you try to diet or reduce caloric intake, the harder LPL works at storing fat. And if you go back to a regular, balanced program of eating, LPL continues storing fat at an increased level.

How to Benefit

It is best to work with LPL rather than against it. Begin by listening to your body—eat when you first sense hunger rather than when you are starving and end up consuming a huge meal. Frequent snacking—every 2 hours, for example—will keep LPL from switching on and storing more fat. Just make certain you are choosing healthy, pH-balancing snacks like celery sticks and almond butter.

Super Health Bonus

Frequent snacking (in contrast to huge meals) not only helps you manage LPL activity; it is also easier on your digestive system and helps keep your blood sugar levels more balanced. To learn more about the miraculous role enzymes play in keeping us healthy and helping us heal from many diseases, check out Tip #20 (page 131) and Tip #33 (page 151).

60-Second Weight-Loss Tip #44:
Eliminate the Microbe That May Be Making You Fat

Eliminating the yeast Candida albicans *helps your body shed weight.*

Did you know that your body may be harboring a microbe that not only defeats your efforts to lose weight but also causes you to gain weight? According to research by Jacob Teitelbaum, MD, at the Fibromyalgia and Fatigue Centers in Dallas, Texas, yeast overgrowth is linked to an average weight gain of 32.5 pounds. That's shocking but true. What's more, according to some estimates, at least 15 million American women suffer from candidiasis—a fungal overgrowth in the intestines. So, getting to the bottom of candidiasis is an important factor in shedding the excess pounds.

At least 150 species of fungi (sometimes called yeasts) are collectively known as candida, but one particular type that frequently tends to become overgrown in the intestines is *Candida albicans.* Candida releases over 80 known toxins that can weaken the body's defenses and cause the mucous membranes of the gut to leak. When the gut becomes leaky, undigested protein molecules pass across the intestinal walls and are absorbed into the bloodstream. This can result in many different health conditions, ranging from allergies to food and chemical sensitivities to autoimmune disorders like fibromyalgia, rheumatoid arthritis, and others.

Fungi or yeast are always present in small amounts in the gut, but they are normally kept in check by good bacteria, or probiotics, in our diet or through supplementation. Now, however, so many factors disrupt the body's natural balance that candidiasis is becoming widespread.

Some of the factors that can lead to candida overgrowth include:

- Alcohol (wine, beer, liquor) intake
- Antibiotic use
- Birth control pills
- Blood sugar imbalances
- Consumption of foods that contain antibiotics and synthetic hormones (nonorganic chicken, dairy products, and meat)

- Excessive sugar intake
- Immunosuppressive drugs (steroids, cortisone, etc.)
- Mercury amalgam dental fillings
- Multiple sexual partners or sex with an infected person
- Nutritional deficiencies
- Poor diet
- Recreational drug use
- Stress, particularly ongoing, chronic stress
- Toxic exposures, especially to mold
- Weakened immunity

Some of the signs and symptoms of candida overgrowth include:

- Acne, psoriasis, eczema, rashes, or hives
- Allergies
- Anal, vaginal, or jock itch
- Anemia
- Anxiety
- Asthma
- Athlete's foot
- Attention deficit disorder (ADD) or attention deficit and hyper-activity disorder (ADHD)
- Autism
- Bloating and flatulence
- Body odor or bad breath
- Brain fog or memory lapses
- Chemical sensitivities
- Constipation or diarrhea
- Cravings for sweets, bread, or alcohol
- Crohn's disease
- Depression
- Difficulty gaining or losing weight

- Diminished libido
- Fatigue that sleep doesn't help
- Fibromyalgia
- Food sensitivities
- Headaches, especially frequent ones
- Heartburn
- Hormonal imbalances
- Hypoglycemia
- Immune dysfunction
- Indecisiveness
- Insomnia
- Irritable bowel syndrome
- Joint or muscle aches
- Lack of concentration
- Mood swings or irritability
- Nasal congestion
- Premenstrual syndrome
- Recurrent bladder, sinus, vaginal yeast, or respiratory infections
- Thyroid conditions
- Unexplained weight changes

This is a long list, and many of the conditions may seem unrelated, but nevertheless, if you have any of the above symptoms or conditions, you may be suffering from candida overgrowth. Of course, other factors may also be present, so you should always contact your physician.

Candida produces hormonelike substances that interfere with normal hormone production. These hormonelike substances can disrupt the body's normal hormone balance, especially in women. Additionally, studies in rats found that candida stimulates histamine production, which is linked to allergic reactions and may cause tissue swelling. Candida overgrowth is likely an underlying factor in some allergic reactions and in the increase in allergies over the past few decades.

Many people are also eating a diet deficient in critical nutrients like vitamins, minerals, amino acids, and essential fatty acids needed to ward off candida infections. Throughout the 60 Seconds to Slim program, you are learning ways to continuously improve your diet to ward off these nutrient deficiencies.

Candidiasis is linked to weight gain in several ways.

- It can interfere with absorption of many critical nutrients needed for detoxification and fat metabolism.

- It triggers intense cravings, particularly for carbohydrates that candida organisms need to live and that allow them to multiply further.

- It interferes with the normal functioning of the thyroid, which reduces the body's ability to convert fat and food into energy needed for cellular functions.

- It causes belly bloating due to the fermentation of carbs and toxic by-products of candida in the intestines.

Many great natural remedies kill candida. Two of my favorites are artemisia and burdock, which cleanse the digestive tract and the blood, respectively.

How to Benefit

Artemisia and burdock are available in capsules or as a tincture (alcohol extract). Follow package instructions.

Some food remedies can also eliminate yeast overgrowth.

- **Garlic.** Just a single clove of raw garlic in your daily diet can shut down the formation of hyphae, the long, branching strands created by yeast to help it grow and spread. Garlic causes the yeast cells to prematurely age and die.[10] Read more about the weight-loss benefits of garlic in Tip #13 on page 120.

- **Coconut Oil.** Research at Nigeria's University College Hospital found that coconut oil kills close to 100 percent of yeast cells (even drug-resistant species) on contact, thanks to its lauric, caprylic, and capric acid content. These ingredients cause the protective outer wall of yeast cells to split apart, making it easier for the immune system to destroy them. Take 3 tablespoons of extra virgin coconut oil daily to obtain the benefits found in the study.[11] (See Tip #19 on page 129 for more information.)

Super Health Bonus

Getting on top of candidiasis not only results in weight loss in most people, but it also improves sinusitis, digestion, immunity, and moods.

60-Second Weight-Loss Tip #45:
Practice Mindful Eating

Eating more slowly and being attentive to what you consume helps you feel full on less food.

Did you know that *how* you eat is as important as *what* you eat when it comes to weight loss? Simply becoming more conscious of how you eat can help you lose weight. Most of us eat on the run, on the road, at our desk, or in front of the television, and often find we don't even remember eating our food. We were too busy with some other task.

To lose more weight, start paying attention to your food habits and do not eat while there are other distractions like work, television, or driving. And eat more slowly. Savor each bite and take your time to completely and thoroughly chew your food. This process of eating more slowly and being more attentive to your eating is called mindfulness eating. It's a type of meditative process that ensures that you don't overeat and that you actually take pleasure in your food. By eating more slowly, you eat less, feel full faster, and enjoy your meals more. And you lose weight.

By eating slowly and practicing mindful eating, you also reduce the chances of overeating because of stress. You will start to see patterns in your eating, such as when you crave specific foods, and become more conscious of the choices you make. When you're stressed out, you may feel more likely to overindulge in chocolate or ice cream. Start to become more aware that you are eating to quell emotions rather than to soothe a growling stomach.

How to Benefit

Start to eat slowly, eliminate distractions while you are eating, and become conscious of chewing and what you're feeling. Stop eating on the run, behind the wheel, or in front of the television. Chew your food thoroughly and completely before swallowing. And stop eating when you feel full, no matter how good the food tastes.

Super Health Bonus

Slowing the pace of eating and being more attentive to eating instead of doing work, watching television, or driving will actually improve your digestion. By focusing your attention on what you're eating and chewing it properly, you are less likely to feel stressed during meals, which means your stress glands will not secrete adrenaline and other stress hormones that take energy away from your digestive organs. Over time, you'll experience improved digestion.

60-Second Weight-Loss Tip #46:
Head Out for a Walk

Walk daily and you can lose 25 pounds in a year—without changing anything else.

Just by making a concerted effort to get off the couch and go for a walk, you can lose 25 pounds this year. Research shows that heading out for a brisk walk or doing some other form of aerobic exercise—the kind that gets you breathing deeper and gets your heart pumping more oxygen—can result in 25 pounds of weight lost in a year, even if you don't change a thing about your diet.[12] That's an incredible amount of weight to lose by simply going for a walk. I'm not suggesting that you don't change your diet. Doing so can increase the amount of weight you can lose, plus eating healthfully is essential to alkalizing your body and attaining a number of other health benefits outlined in this book.

If walking outdoors is not for you, you can reap the same benefits on a treadmill or stationary bike or by doing another type of brisk activity. Any exercise that gets you breathing deeper works.

How to Benefit

There's no fancy equipment needed, no designer gear, and no special techniques to learn to benefit from this research. All you have to do is motivate yourself to get moving. And do it daily. Find a time that works well for you and stick to it every day or at least 5 days a week. Maybe walking home from work instead of driving is best for you. Or perhaps heading outdoors for a walk after dinner. Taking the stairs instead of the elevator is also good if you have enough floors in your office building or home. Whatever works for you that you'll also stick with is the best approach.

Super Health Bonus

You'll boost lung and heart function. By getting your blood pumping harder and by breathing deeper, you'll oxygenate your blood, which oxygenates every cell and tissue in your body, but especially your lungs and heart.

60-Second Weight-Loss Tip #47:
Add Resistance Training

Resistance training, like weight lifting, results in a 73 percent increase in fat burning for hours afterward.

Just adding 15 to 20 minutes of resistance training like lifting weights results in a 73 percent increase in fat burning for hours after you finish, according to research at the University of Nevada. Resistance training helps to build lean muscle, which is more compact than fat, and helps to ramp up your fat-burning efforts.[13] Even lifting 5-pound weights helps you to get this impressive result and develop great muscle tone.

Hopefully you have been doing some kind of cardio exercise for the past few weeks on the program. Here's a smart timing trick that can help you get the most out of both types of workout and also help you avoid mindless eating: In one study, people who walked for 15 minutes, then did 15 minutes of muscle-toning exercise, ate 517 fewer calories per day than those who just walked or just did strength training.[14] It seems that the combination of walking immediately followed by strength training makes you feel less hungry. It also helps build muscles that bolster your metabolism to burn fat around the clock.

How to Benefit

If you don't already have weights, you can purchase some 5-pound weights or use some heavy canned goods. Even lifting bags of groceries in different

ways while you're watching television is a good weight-training option.
If you can afford to join a gym, that's great, but don't let the lack of a gym
membership or weight equipment be an excuse not to exercise.

A number of moves can help you reap these benefits. You learned a
few good ones in The Essential Plan. Flip back to page 80 for a refresher.
Many fitness magazines and online sources have additional strength-
training ideas, and if you do belong to a gym, the staff members are a
valuable resource.

Super Health Bonus

Correctly lifting weights helps improve structural integrity and balance,
which can result in reduced likelihood of injury or pain.

60-Second Weight-Loss Tip #48:
Visualize Yourself Thin

*Think yourself thin by taking a few moments to visualize what you'll look like when
you reach your desired weight.*

Here's a surprisingly simple exercise to lose weight that doesn't involve
cardio or weights or even getting off the couch: visualization. That's right.
Thinking yourself thin may be one of the best, yet least used, exercises for
weight loss.

According to a study in the *Journal of Consulting and Clinical Psychology*,
people who used guided imagery were significantly more likely to keep
weight off for good than those who didn't use this simple process.[15] "What
is guided imagery?" you may be asking. It's as simple as picturing how you
will look when you lose excess weight, along with imagining how you will
feel. The more you can visualize yourself and feel the emotions involved,
the greater the chances of losing the weight and keeping it off.

The study found that even just taking a minute or two each day to imagine
the things you will do, the compliments you will hear, the way you will feel,
and the energy you'll experience can have a significant effect. And not only
does it help keep weight off, but researchers found that it has other benefits
as well. One hundred percent of people who used guided visualization found

it easier to stick to their weight-loss program. Scientists also found that it boosted motivation and prevented stress eating. According to one study, binge eating dropped by 74 percent among people who practiced this simple exercise on a daily basis.

What's more, simply imagining yourself using weights can actually tone your muscles and improve your strength. The Cleveland Clinic asked study participants to visualize themselves exercising specific muscles, without actually working out these muscle groups. In just 12 weeks researchers found that the participants had increased muscle strength by 13 percent without having lifted a single weight.[16]

Don't get me wrong. I'm not suggesting that you skip the exercise in favor of imagery, but it's hard to make excuses for not visualizing yourself exercising. Not enough energy? No time? It's just so simple that even these excuses don't work.

How to Benefit

While sitting, standing, or lying down, close your eyes for a moment and visualize your body at your optimum weight. How does your abdomen look? What about your hips and thighs? Try to get as much detail in your picture of your ideal body as possible. Imagine yourself feeling confident and energetic, doing all the things you love to do and maybe even some things you've never done but always wanted to. How does it feel? What emotions do you experience?

Then, visualize a part of your body you'd especially like to tone. Picture yourself lifting weights with this body part and see yourself getting stronger and stronger. Imagine the muscles actually looking fit and toned. Experience your body as powerful and strong. How do you feel?

Try to stay in the visualization for at least a minute, preferably two or three. But, even if you only have a minute, you can benefit from this simple visualization exercise. And it can be done almost anywhere: at your desk, while walking (with your eyes open, of course), during a commercial break while watching television, before you get out of bed in the morning, or just as you retire in the evening.

Super Health Bonus

Using guided visualization on a regular basis not only keeps you motivated, helps keep the weight off, improves muscle strength and tone, and reduces the likelihood of binge eating; it also can improve your health. Research shows it helps reduce pain and fight illness too.

60-Second Weight-Loss Tip #49:
Address Emotional Issues

Learn how to release your pent-up negative emotions linked with excess weight.

Let's face it: We all have emotional issues, so it should come as no surprise that weight gain can be linked to them. The issues can be almost anything: fear, anger, feeling vulnerable or not good enough, or being out of harmony with our true self, among others.

Research by neuroscientist Candace Pert even shows that we store emotions in the cells of our bodies.[17] That's why many people start to feel emotional issues rise to the surface as they lose weight. When you slim down, fat cells do not just lose fat. They're also losing pent-up emotions. If you've ever had a great massage or other form of bodywork, followed by an emotional release after a trauma or other stressful occurrence in your life, you're probably already aware of how your whole body holds on to emotions. Successful weight loss means finding an outlet to release those stresses from your body. There are many ways to do that.

How to Benefit

Here are some ways to help you cope with the emotions that may be an underlying factor in your weight issues.

- **Crying.** Sometimes simply allowing yourself some alone time to cry can lift the weight off your shoulders—and the rest of you.

- **Running or jogging.** Many people find that running or jogging is a great way to release emotions. The exercise releases endorphins, and there's lots of time to clear your mind when it's just you and the road (or the treadmill).

- **Singing.** After I had a spinal cord injury and could no longer run, I discovered that cranking up the music and singing was a fantastic release of emotions. If you need alone time to do it, tell the people with whom you live that you need some time for yourself. Most people will understand.

- **Meditating.** Just get comfortable and, whenever thoughts come to mind, move them aside. Eventually, you'll get good at simply "being."

- **Energy medicine.** Here's an excellent energy medicine technique: Lie down in a comfortable place. Think about some issue that is troubling you. Allow yourself to truly feel the pain, frustration, fear, or whatever feeling you're having. While doing this, hold your hand across your forehead. When we are upset the blood in our brain moves to the back of the head to a part of our brain that is sometimes called the "dinosaur brain" because it is fairly primitive. Holding your hand across the front of your forehead gives off heat, electromagnetic and infrared energy that brings blood back to the front of the brain, allowing our brain to think of clearer solutions and allowing our emotions to be healed and released. This may take a few minutes or it may take 10 to 20 minutes. The more you can feel the emotional pain during this time, the more effective the healing tends to be.

- **Writing.** Write out your issues. One of the things I find particularly helpful is to write without censorship. That means taking some time for yourself when you're feeling awful and just writing whatever comes to mind. Don't worry whether it is politically correct or if you're using words you normally wouldn't say. Allow yourself the freedom to express exactly what you feel, and release it. I usually find a safe spot to burn these pages afterward to fully release them. After all, storing these emotions by keeping these pages just prevents you from fully releasing them from your being.

Super Health Bonus

Not only will dealing with underlying emotions help your weight-loss efforts, but it will also help you to feel more confident and strong. Sometimes just releasing these emotions in a healthy way can help you to feel less burdened by them, freeing up more energy to feel great.

60-Second Weight-Loss Tip #50:
Support Your Stress Glands

The following techniques reverse damage to the stress glands and balance the hormones that cause weight gain.

If the pace of life has left you frazzled or if balancing work, home, and family responsibilities has left you overwhelmed, your stress glands may be overworked. The stresses of our modern life can be too much for these glands to handle. The stress glands, primarily known as the adrenal glands, are two small, triangular glands that sit atop the kidneys. We don't give them much thought until we start to experience symptoms of poor health, low energy, or weight gain, particularly abdominal fat.

The adrenal glands keep us going through life's stresses, but over time they can show signs of being overworked. When they are overworked, they secrete excess cortisol that signals your body that you might be in serious trouble so it should hold on to any fat you have. This mechanism worked beautifully when your ancient ancestors were on the run from bears or had difficulty finding sufficient food. But given today's lifestyles, the same mechanism causes us to become overweight.

How do you know if your adrenal glands are working too hard? Here are 25 signs that they may be overworked.

1. Allergies
2. Anxiety or irritability
3. Arthritis
4. Cravings for salty and/or sweet foods
5. Depression
6. Excessive hunger
7. Extreme fatigue, exhaustion, or chronic fatigue
8. Feeling of being overwhelmed or unable to cope with life's stresses
9. Frequent colds, flus, or other infections
10. Insomnia
11. Irritable bowel syndrome (IBS)
12. Low blood pressure

13. Low libido

14. Low stamina

15. Menopause symptoms (hot flashes, mood swings, vaginal dryness)

16. Poor concentration

17. Poor digestion

18. Premenstrual syndrome

19. Reduced immune function

20. Reduced memory

21. Sensitivity to cold

22. Sensitivity to light

23. Sleep that does not refresh or revitalize you

24. Slow recovery from illness or injuries

25. Weight gain, particularly abdominal weight gain

These symptoms can also be signs of other health conditions, so you should always consult your doctor if you suspect any health issues. And, of course, you don't need to be experiencing all of the above symptoms to be suffering from adrenal fatigue.

In short-term stressful situations, the adrenal glands' output of hormones such as adrenaline and cortisol may be beneficial, helping us to cope with the stress. But over time, dealing with chronic stresses depletes these organs and makes us prone to weight gain, exhaustion, and other health problems. There are many ways to rebalance the adrenal glands, but the best way is to make efforts to reduce stress.

Additionally, find ways to handle stress so it doesn't impact your body negatively. Of course, if you suspect severe adrenal gland problems, you should always consult your physician, since such issues can be life threatening. Here are some ways to restore adrenal gland health. By now, you should already be doing some of them, but if you suspect adrenal gland fatigue as a cause of your belly fat or other fat, you might want to add some additional strategies to your program.

How to Benefit

Here are 14 ways to help strengthen your adrenal glands. You don't need to do all of them, but you can if you want to. Otherwise, pick the ones that feel right for you. In my experience, most people gravitate toward the easiest ones, not necessarily the ones they most need. So be honest with yourself. If one of the items sounds difficult to you, it may be because it's exactly what you need.

1. **Give fast food a break.** You should already be doing this, but an occasional reminder never hurts. Usually loaded with neurotoxins like monosodium glutamate (MSG), fast food can cause your body to be in a constant state of stress after eating it, until the chemicals are detoxified from your system. Depending on the strength of your liver's detoxification systems, that can be anywhere from a few hours to several days.

2. **Take a deep breath . . . and then take a few more.** Research shows that even a few minutes of deep breathing can have an impact on the adrenal glands by reducing the stress hormones they secrete. Instead of jumping out of your seat during a traffic jam or other stressful situation, start breathing deeply.

3. **Reduce your stress.** Okay, I know this sounds impossible to many people. But the truth is that no one else is going to reduce your stress. While life can be stressful sometimes, it's important to take some time on a daily basis to release stress. Go for a walk, stop and smell the roses (literally), give a loved one a hug, practice meditation, get some rest, or practice some other form of stress management.

4. **Eat plentiful amounts of fresh fruits and vegetables.** You should definitely be doing this one by now, but if you aren't, now is the time to add more veggies (and a few fruits) to your diet. Chronic stress depletes nutrients. By eating a diet rich in nutrients from fresh fruit and vegetables, you'll give your body the vitamins, minerals, and phytonutrients that help it recover.

5. **Reduce your caffeine intake.** Caffeine stimulates the adrenal glands, only to cause an energy crash later on. Try herbal teas instead. Peppermint tea is a natural pick-me-up that doesn't stimulate the adrenal glands.

6. **Try to get at least 7 or 8 hours of sleep at night.** And if possible, don't wake to a blaring alarm clock since the noise causes a flood of stress hormones to be released.

7. **Practice the yoga posture Viparita Karani.** For those of you who don't speak Sanskrit (myself included), that means "legs up the wall." While keeping your legs up the wall, elevate your pelvis on a bolster or folded blankets. According to yoga expert Roger Cole, "If the legs tire of being straight, bend the knees and cross the legs, with knees near the wall." According to Cole, "This pose stimulates baroreceptors [blood pressure sensors] in the neck and upper chest, triggering reflexes that reduce nerve input into the adrenal glands, slow the heart rate, slow the brain waves, relax blood vessels, and reduce the amount of norepinephrine circulating in the bloodstream."

8. **Exercise regularly but don't overdo it.** Exercise is a valuable release for pent-up stresses. Just know your limits and don't overexercise, since it can cause stress on the adrenals.

9. **Take some vitamin C.** The adrenal glands use more vitamin C than any other organ or gland in the body. Vitamin C is essential to manufacture adrenal gland hormones. So when you've been chronically stressed, your adrenals may have depleted your vitamin C stores. A typical daily dose to assist with adrenal stress is 500 to 2,000 milligrams or higher—higher doses may be necessary in extreme cases. Of course, a qualified health professional should be consulted when using higher doses or before taking any new supplements.

10. **Take some extra vitamin B$_5$.** Also known as pantothenic acid, B$_5$ is necessary for adrenal gland health. While it is naturally present in the adrenal glands, it can become depleted as hormones are manufactured in response to stress. A common daily dose for adrenal fatigue is 1,500 milligrams, but it should always accompany a B-complex vitamin since these nutrients work synergistically.

11. **Avoid sugar and refined wheat products.** They cause your blood sugar to fluctuate rapidly, which in turn causes your adrenals to overreact. Again, this is something you should already be doing, but if you aren't, this is added incentive to move your diet onto the right track.

12. **Eat some protein at every meal.** Protein stabilizes blood sugar and prevents strain on the adrenals. That doesn't necessarily mean meat. As I mentioned earlier, some good vegetarian sources of protein include legumes (beans), nuts, seeds, avocado, and quinoa (a delicious whole grain).

13. **Supplement with Siberian ginseng.** Depending on how serious your adrenal stress may be, you may also benefit from herbal support from *Eleutherococcus senticosus,* as it is also known. It works primarily on the pituitary gland in the brain to better regulate adrenal gland function. In adrenal fatigue, communication between the pituitary gland and the adrenals may be impaired. A typical dose of Siberian ginseng for the treatment of adrenal fatigue is 100 to 200 milligrams daily.

14. **Take a page from Ayurveda.** Practitioners of Ayurvedic medicine— the Indian form of natural medicine with a several-thousand-year-old history—recommend ashwagandha, or *Withania somnifera,* as it is also known. Ashwagandha is a tonic for fatigue and exhaustion, memory loss, muscle weakness, and other symptoms of adrenal fatigue. It can normalize adrenal gland hormones. One to 2 teaspoons of an ashwagandha tincture daily is the commonly recommended dose. Always consult your physician prior to use.

Super Health Bonus

Boosting your adrenal gland function will strengthen your immune system, significantly bolster your energy levels, and help you to just feel better over- all. These glands play such an important role in your body's health that giv- ing them the support they need can make a difference in almost any health issue you're experiencing.

60-Second Weight-Loss Tip #51:
Adopt Liver-Boosting Strategies

Heal fatty liver disease, an underlying health condition that could be making you fat.
     Your liver is one of the most important weight-loss organs. Located under your lower ribs on the right side of your abdomen, your liver is responsible for over 500 functions, including eliminating excess hormones, detoxifying harmful chemicals that would otherwise be stored in fat reposi- tories on your body, creating the thousands of enzymes that control virtually

every function of your body, and breaking down fat. Your liver is arguably one of the most overworked organs in your body.

The liver also secretes a substance called bile that is stored in the gallbladder. The liver metabolizes proteins, fats, and carbohydrates.

Thanks to our modern lifestyle, the liver has more than its fair share of work. Every foreign substance that enters your body must be filtered by your liver. These include alcohol; tobacco; environmental pollutants; food additives; pesticides; common cosmetic ingredients; household products; stress hormones or excess sex, thyroid, or adrenal hormones; pharmaceutical and over-the-counter drugs; caffeine; and many more.

And with the average person consuming 14 pounds of food preservatives, additives, waxes, colorings, flavors, antimicrobials, and pesticide residues in her food annually, her liver must devote significant energy to detoxifying them and/or removing them from the body.[18] Your liver must filter every medication you take, including commonly used antibiotics and acetaminophen, sometimes resulting in damage to this important organ. And, of course, your liver must filter every alcoholic beverage you drink. So you can imagine how critical it is in our modern age of chemical exposure to keep your liver functioning as efficiently as possible.

If you're one of the millions of people who've tried low-fat diets, your liver may be suffering from nutritional deficiencies that result in slower fat and toxin metabolism. On this type of diet, the body does not obtain sufficient essential fatty acids, which are the building blocks of a healthy metabolism, immune system, hormonal system, and more. Forget weight loss on a low- fat diet; more likely, you'll gain health problems.

While the liver can continue working even when it has lost up to 80 percent of its ability to function, there is a significant difference between functioning and optimal functioning. When it comes to weight loss, we're concerned with boosting the liver's function for peak performance. Fortunately, the liver has an incredible capacity for regeneration.

How do you know if your liver is functioning well? Of course, your doctor can order medical tests, but they primarily show poor liver health when it's fairly advanced. You can learn a lot about your liver's health by assessing whether you have signs of liver stress. Take the following quiz to determine whether you might be suffering from reduced liver function, liver toxicity, or a fatty liver.

Do you experience any of the following?

- Abdominal bloating
- Alcohol intolerance
- Allergies
- Asthma
- Bad breath or a coated tongue
- Bowel infections
- Brain "fog"
- Chronic fatigue syndrome
- Cravings for sweets
- Crohn's disease
- Dark circles under the eyes
- Depression
- Difficulty losing weight
- Environmental illness or multiple chemical sensitivities
- Fatigue
- Fevers
- Fibromyalgia
- Fluid retention
- Gallbladder disease
- Gallstones or gravel (in the gallbladder)
- Gastritis
- Headaches and migraines
- Hepatitis
- High blood pressure
- High cholesterol levels
- Hives
- Hormone imbalances
- Hypoglycemia (unstable blood sugar levels)
- Immune system disorders
- Indigestion
- Irritable bowel syndrome

- Mood swings
- Overweight or obesity
- Poor appetite
- Poor digestion
- Recurring nausea and/or vomiting with no known cause
- Skin diseases
- Slow metabolism
- Ulcerative colitis

If you are suffering from any of these symptoms or conditions, you may benefit from strengthening your liver's ability to detoxify and metabolize fats.[19] You can learn more about fatty liver disease in Tip #14 on page 121.

How to Benefit

Here are liver-boosting strategies you can incorporate into your program (if you aren't using them already) to ensure your liver is getting the support it needs to help you shed pounds.

1. Since the liver requires high amounts of vitamins and minerals to perform its many functions, your diet should be high in fruits and vegetables and nutrient-rich foods. You're probably doing this already, but if not, now is the time to add more veggies and a few fruits to your diet.

2. Because food additives and preservatives need to be filtered by your liver, your diet should be free of processed foods, artificial food additives, colors, and preservatives to take the load off your liver. Additionally, choose to eat a diet low in refined sugar and synthetic sweeteners.

3. You should definitely be avoiding margarine, shortening, and commercial oils. Instead, choose unrefined oils from the refrigerator section of your local health food store. Avoid eating animal fat and fried foods as well.

4. Drink 1 quart or liter per 50 pounds of current body weight of water every day. This is the only way your liver can flush toxins out of your body.

5. Better yet, start every day with a large glass of water with the fresh juice of one-half to one lemon added. Lemon helps bolster your liver's detoxification abilities. Drink the remaining daily water with pH drops. Don't use lemon juice and pH drops in the same glass of water.

6. Eat plenty of liver-rebuilding foods, including carrots, beets, leafy greens, and other green vegetables.

7. Eat lots of garlic, onions, and broccoli since these foods contain the sulfur that is required to increase the liver's detoxification ability.

8. Your liver's detoxification efforts require considerable amounts of nutrients to function properly, so be sure to take a high-quality multivitamin and mineral supplement. Even a single nutrient deficiency can seriously disrupt natural detoxification processes.

9. While lying flat on your back, you can gently massage the liver/gallbladder area, which is located along the lower rib on the right side of your body. This helps improve circulation to the area.

10. Some excellent herbs help your liver rebuild. Here are some of my preferred ones. There's no need to take all of them—one or two will usually be sufficient. All are excellent options; be sure to follow manufacturers' directions.

   - Burdock root
   - Dandelion root
   - Milk thistle seed
   - Turmeric root

Super Health Bonus

Rebuilding the liver will dramatically boost your ability to detoxify excess hormones and toxins, helping to restore hormonal balance to your body. It will even help to improve your digestion.

60-Second Weight-Loss Tip #52:
Eat Breakfast

Eighty percent of overweight people skip breakfast. Eat breakfast and dramatically improve weight loss.

People trying to lose weight often think that eating less and skipping meals is the best way to drop pounds, but studies show that simply isn't the case. According to research, eating breakfast is far more likely to cause you to lose weight than skipping this essential meal.

Eating breakfast helps restore blood sugar balance after a night of not eating, hence the name, "break fast." Your body fasts during the night while you sleep, and when you wake up, it needs food. Eating within 1 hour of waking is critical to signal to your body that you aren't starving and it doesn't need to hoard fat. Doing so allows the body to start breaking down fat stores.

How to Benefit

It's fairly easy to benefit from this important research. Simply start eating breakfast. Don't have time? Prepare a healthy breakfast the night before. It could be as simple as cooking extra quinoa at dinner and warming it in the morning with a little almond milk. Or drink an almond milk, fruit, and greens smoothie that can be whipped up in a minute in a blender. And if you have one of the many personal blenders available, the canisters are usually travel containers as well. So there really is no excuse for skipping breakfast. I have provided an assortment of slimming breakfast recipes you can try, beginning on page 237.

Super Health Bonus

Eating breakfast helps to provide the fuel your body and brain need to function properly throughout the day. You'll experience a boost in energy and brainpower just by eating breakfast every day.

60-Second Weight-Loss Tip #53:
Breathe Deeply to Halt Fat-Gaining Hormones

Breathing deeply reduces stress hormones linked to weight gain in seconds.

We often think that something must be difficult or intensive to burn fat. But, that's not true. Simply breathing more deeply can help you lose weight. I know, it sounds surprising, but it works. Deep breathing helps your body regulate stress hormones, like cortisol, that are linked to weight gain. It works in two ways.

1. Within 60 seconds, it sends signals to your brain to relax your nervous system, which tells your adrenals to stop pumping out cortisol. They normally do this to help your body deal with stress, but when stresses start to become chronic, so does the cortisol—and that causes your body to hoard fat, particularly abdominal fat. When you breathe deeply, your body quickly starts to relax, signaling that the stress is over and that it should cutt off the production of cortisol. When you continue to practice deep-breathing exercises, you shut off chronic overproduction of fat-hoarding cortisol.

2. Deep breathing also increases oxygen levels in your bloodstream, which gives you more energy. In a study of cyclists, researchers found that those who practiced deep breathing could cycle 50 percent farther than usual. Deep breathing can increase your endurance, helping you to walk farther or last longer during your exercise sessions. Even small increases in exercise can add up to big weight loss.[28]

How to Benefit

Try this simple deep-breathing exercise: Sit, stand, or lie down in a comfortable position while maintaining good posture. Gently take a slightly deeper breath than you normally do, but don't force it—it should feel natural and comfortable. Hold the breath slightly without straining. Exhale. Gently take a deeper breath into the diaphragm region of your upper abdomen; you should feel your stomach rising as you inhale and lowering as you exhale. Hold slightly and then exhale, being sure to exhale fully. Repeat for at least a minute but longer if you have the time. Try to perform this simple breathing exercise periodically throughout the day. You can do it while sitting at work, waiting to see your doctor, or taking a stroll. While it's a good idea to take some deep breaths when driving to ease the stress of commuting, traffic congestion, or road rage, be sure to keep your eyes open and maintain alertness.

And remember, try to keep your posture straight. When you slouch, you compress your lungs, lowering the amount of air, and therefore oxygen, you inhale. Straight posture while sitting or standing helps maximize the amount of oxygen you breathe, increasing the energizing and cortisol-lowering benefits you reap. Exhausted? It's okay to lie down to perform a few minutes of deep breathing.

Super Health Bonus

Breathing deeply, but still in a natural, unforced way oxygenates your blood, which in turn alkalizes your body. You'll experience a calm state of energy.

60-Second SUCCESS STORY

Maria Newcomer

Age: **45**
Location: **New Bedford, MA**
Occupation: **Early childhood educator**

Total Weight Lost:
13 pounds

Total Inches Lost:
7.75

> "My clothes fit so much better."

How I Got Here:

Maria Newcomer was feeling frustrated, heavy, and exhausted. "I first heard about Dr. Michelle 3 years ago when I read her book *The Ultimate pH Solution,* and that's when I became very interested in learning more about improving my conditions by eating a more alkaline diet." She was beset with serious asthma attacks every 6 to 8 weeks and was being prescribed steroids and antibiotics to control them. Reducing the factors that heightened the severity of her asthma attacks was what motivated her. "I wanted to learn better nutrition, feel better, have more energy, improve my health, and control the asthma by eating alkaline foods." Her first challenge? She needed to face her Pepsi-drinking and candy-eating habits head on.

(continued)

Progress Report:

Maria shares: "I was thrilled to lose weight and inches. Most of all, though, I was encouraged by the fact that my asthma symptoms seemed to decrease while following the program, which was a *big* motivation factor for me!"

Beyond:

Since starting 60 Seconds to Slim, Maria says, "I now have more energy throughout the day. No more energy slumps or naps in the middle of the day! My health and asthma have improved so I'm feeling better."

Prior to her starting the program, Maria's shirt size was a 16/18 and a month later she's down to a 14/16. "I was very pleased to lose several pounds and inches on this program. I intend to continue following it and losing even more weight and inches." Maria adds: "I feel much better, so I have more of a positive outlook on life!"

After a very positive month on the program, she plans to keep up the good work. "I will be learning better nutrition, experimenting with recipes, decreasing the inflammation in my body, increasing my exercise level, and working on continuing to improve my asthma."

Chapter 6

Week 4: SUPPLEMENT

Use These Supplements to Dissolve Fat

This week you will learn about proven weight-loss nutrients and remedies, how to supplement your diet with them, which ones to choose for their specific metabolic properties, and how these remedies can dramatically increase your body's ability to burn fat while improving your health.

And don't worry, you won't have to take all the remedies outlined in this section. Choose two that sound like a good fit for you, in light of any health issues or specific challenges to weight loss that you might be experiencing. Some of the tips will include questionnaires to help you decide whether you may be suffering from an underlying hormonal or glandular imbalance that can be rectified with natural remedies. Here are the 60-Second Weight-Loss Tips you'll learn this week:

54. Take Two Phytonutrients (page 207)
> *Resveratrol and isoflavones cause fat cells to self-destruct.*

55. Add Quercetin to Dissolve Stubborn Fat (page 209)
> *In addition to resveratrol and isoflavones, adding quercetin creates a phytonutrient cocktail that packs a fat-fighting punch.*

56. Smell Your Way Thin (page 210)
> *Enjoy the blissful blend of aromatherapy oils that causes a significant drop in abdominal fat.*

57. Shrink Fat Cells with Chromium (page 212)
> *The mineral chromium is proven to suppress the hormones linked to fat cell expansion.*

58. Supplement with Fat to Lose Fat (page 214)
> *Omega-3 fatty acids turn off your fat genes and increase the fat burned during exercise by 14 percent.*

59. Inhale Vanilla to Stop Cravings (page 215)
> *Inhaling the natural scent of vanilla can cause you to lose 5 pounds in 4 weeks without even trying.*

60. Take Bacteria to Transform Your Body's Inner Workings (page 217)
> *Supplementing with probiotics transforms your inner terrain to that of a thin person.*

61. Supplement with Calcium to Neutralize Acid (page 221)
> *Calcium is a superalkaline mineral that neutralizes acid to boost your weight loss.*

62. Take Grape Seed Extract to Stop Belly Fat Formation (page 223)
> *Grape seed extract is proven to stop the formation of belly fat in its tracks.*

63. Take Carnitine to Burn Fat Fast (page 224)

> *Carnitine is a powerful nutrient that transports fat to your cells'*
> *incinerators to be burned as fuel.*

64. Mop Up Free Fadicals with Lipoic Acid (page 226)

> *Lipoic acid is a powerful antioxidant that mops up free radicals linked to*
> *inflammation, weight gain, and disease.*

65. Detoxify More Fat with Natural Herbs (page 227)

> *Milk thistle, dandelion, globe artichoke, and turmeric boost your liver's*
> *ability to break down harmful fats, excessive hormones, and toxins linked to*
> *weight gain.*

60-Second Weight-Loss Tip #54:
Take Two Phytonutrients

Resveratrol and isoflavones cause fat cells to self-destruct.

A potent phytonutrient combination found in certain common foods actually causes fat cells to self-destruct! This exciting new research, led by MaryAnne Della-Fera, PhD, at the University of Georgia, identified an all-natural nutrient cocktail that works on the body in two ways to significantly assist with weight loss. First, it reduces cells' ability to store fat by about 130 percent, and second, it causes fat cells to disintegrate at a rate 246 percent higher than normal. What is this powerful food combination? After numerous attempts to identify the most potent nutrient fat-burning cocktail, Dr. Della-Fera learned that isoflavones found in soy foods and resveratrol found in grapes caused the greatest fat-burning effect. Participants in her study experienced weight losses of between 4 and 10 pounds per week.[1]

The liver is the body's main fat-digesting organ. Every molecule of fat that you eat must pass through your liver, but if your liver is overburdened by its more than 500 other essential activities, it can become sluggish. The combination of isoflavones and resveratrol seems to strengthen the detoxification pathways in the liver and supercharge its ability to break down fat. The result is a stronger, healthier liver that breaks down fat in your body.

How to Benefit

Isoflavones and resveratrol can be obtained from foods. Isoflavones are found in soy foods, including soy milk, tofu, miso (a fermented soybean paste commonly used to make soups and salad dressings), edamame, natto (a fermented, cooked soy product), soy flour, soy yogurt, soy nuts, soy nut butter, soy sprouts, and tempeh. Resveratrol is found in purple and red grapes, purple grape juice, red wine, berries, and cherries.

While you can get these phytonutrients in foods, Dr. Della-Fera obtained the best results when people supplemented their diet with 100 milligrams each of isoflavones and resveratrol in pill form, both readily available in most health food stores. You can expect the same results Dr. Della-Fera achieved by supplementing with the same dose.

Take both supplements at once. If you experience nausea, simply cut back your daily dose to 25 milligrams each of isoflavones and resveratrol and add 25 milligrams more of each nutrient each week until you get to the 100-milligram dose.

To obtain more isoflavones in your diet, drink 1 to 2 cups of organic soy milk daily and eat MSG-free miso soup three to four times per week. Many restaurants claim their miso soup is free of MSG, but they may still be using ingredients such as chicken base or soy sauce that contain the harmful ingredient.

Safety Consideration

Avoid taking isoflavones if you are at high risk of breast cancer or have a soy allergy.

Super Health Bonus

Isoflavones have been shown in studies to lessen the difficult symptoms many women face during the menopausal years, particularly hot flashes.

Research shows that resveratrol protects brain cells from free radical damage linked to brain diseases, including Alzheimer's disease.

60-Second Weight-Loss Tip #55:
Add Quercetin to Dissolve Stubborn Fat

In addition to resveratrol and isoflavones, adding quercetin creates a phytonutrient cocktail that packs a fat-fighting punch.

Recent research in the *Journal of Medicinal Food* found that adding one additional nutrient to Dr. Mary Anne Della-Fera's phytonutrient weight-loss combination (see Tip #54 on page 207) further increases its ability to burn fat. Dr. Hea Jin Park and colleagues at the University of Georgia found that the natural isoflavone genistein—a particular type of isoflavone—from soy and resveratrol from purple grapes worked even better when quercetin was added to the mix.

Recall that Dr. Della-Fera found that resveratrol and isoflavones cause fat cells to self-destruct. Dr. Park and colleagues showed that adding quercetin was even more effective. The scientists examined the ability of genistein, resveratrol, and quercetin in combination and alone to increase fat burning and reduce fat accumulation. They found the combination was substantially more effective than the nutrients were on their own.[2]

In addition to the anti-inflammatory effects of resveratrol and the hormone-balancing effects of isoflavones, quercetin helps reduce inflammation and allergic reactions that cause swelling and weight gain.

How to Benefit

Supplement with 100 milligrams each of isoflavones (the study focused on the isoflavone genistein), resveratrol, and quercetin. You can also obtain these phytonutrients from foods. Isoflavones are found in soy foods, including soy milk, tofu, miso (a fermented soybean paste commonly used to make soups and salad dressings), edamame, natto (a fermented, cooked soy product), soy flour, soy yogurt, soy nuts, soy nut butter, soy sprouts, and tempeh. Resveratrol is found in purple and red grapes, purple grape juice, red wine, berries, and cherries. Quercetin is found in onions and apples.

Super Health Bonus

The addition of quercetin to your diet can alleviate inflammation linked to allergies, reducing seasonal allergy symptoms like runny or stuffy nose, and watery or itchy eyes.

60-Second Weight-Loss Tip #56:
Smell Your Way Thin

Enjoy the blissful blend of aromatherapy oils that causes a significant drop in abdominal fat.

Exciting research at the Department of Nursing at the Wonkwang Health Science College in Korea reveals that aromatherapy abdominal massage can reduce belly fat. The scientists divided postmenopausal women into two groups. All study participants massaged their own abdomen twice daily for 5 days each week for 6 weeks. One group used only grape seed oil, while the other groups used a blend of grapefruit, lemon, and cypress essential oils.

The scientists found that the women who used the essential oil blend had significantly less abdominal fat at the end of the 6-week study. Additionally, their waist measurements also dropped significantly and they experienced a significant improvement in body image compared with the grape seed oil control group. (To find out how you can supplement with grape seed oil to lose weight, however, check out Tip #62 on page 223.) These results suggest that aromatherapy massage with grapefruit, cypress, and lemon oils is an excellent way to aid the loss of belly fat. While the study involved only postmenopausal women, it is likely that the same results would be found in others too.

Additional research from Niigata University School of Medicine in Japan showed that grapefruit and lemon oils activated the body's ability to burn fat and suppress any further weight gain.[3]

How to Benefit

Here's how to make a bottle of abdominal fat–busting massage oil.

1. Measure 2 ounces of sweet almond oil in a glass measuring cup. (Sweet almond oil acts as a carrier oil for the grapefruit, lemon, and cypress essential oils.)
2. Add 5 drops each of pure grapefruit, lemon, and cypress essential oils to the measuring cup.
3. Pour into a glass bottle with a lid, put the lid on, and shake to blend all ingredients together.
4. Use a small amount of the oil blend to massage your abdomen daily—or twice daily for best results.

Massage technique: Rub the oil in large circles starting above your belly button, working the oil out to the left side of your abdomen, downward and across the lower part of your abdomen, and back up the right side of your abdomen.

Participants in the study conducted abdominal massage with these oils five times a week, so that is the minimum amount recommended to see results; however, you can do it every day if you'd like.

Safety Consideration

Avoid using the oil just prior to sun exposure on the area since grapefruit and lemon oils can cause slight photosensitivity. Wait at least a few hours. Avoid using if you are pregnant or nursing. Discontinue use if you observe any rashes, hives, or other sign of an allergic reaction.

Super Health Bonus

Abdominal massage improves circulation to all the organs housed in that region of your body, including the intestines, liver, pancreas, gallbladder, stomach, and bladder. Improved circulation to these organs helps them to function better. What's more, both grapefruit oil and cypress oil improve mood by reducing depression and anxiety. Cypress is also used by aromatherapists to help people deal with grief and other emotionally difficult times. By massaging in large circles, you'll also help your colon move toxins out of your body.

60-Second Weight-Loss Tip #57:
Shrink Fat Cells with Chromium

The mineral chromium is proved to suppress the hormones linked to fat cell expansion.

As you learned earlier, when your blood sugar surges, your insulin levels rise too, and that can cause your body to hoard fat, making it difficult to lose weight. Combine that with a chromium deficiency and you're at risk for being overweight or obese or becoming diabetic. Some experts estimate that over 90 percent of North Americans are deficient in the mineral chromium, largely because of agricultural practices that deplete the soil and food-manufacturing processes that eradicate chromium and other minerals. Yet this mineral can help restore insulin balance and promote weight loss.

Insulin resistance—or metabolic syndrome—is common in people who are overweight. This is a condition in which the hormone insulin becomes less effective at reducing blood sugar levels. When blood sugar levels stay unnaturally high, the result is often weight gain and a tendency toward diabetes. The mineral chromium helps prevent and reverse insulin resistance, stabilizes blood sugar levels, and allows your cells to function more effectively.

Research at the University of Texas found that supplementing with the mineral chromium daily can help you double fat loss without losing muscle.[4] Chromium helps ensure proper sensitivity to insulin, the hormone secreted by your pancreas to escort sugar to the cells where it is needed before it can damage organs or be converted into fat.

While an important mineral, chromium is often overlooked. It helps maintain strong artery, blood, and heart health, and it also plays a significant role in alleviating a "sweet tooth." Chromium lessens cravings, mood swings, and weight gain linked to fluctuating blood sugar levels since it helps to keep them balanced. Chromium also plays an important role in energy production in our bodies.

When sugarcane is processed to make sugar, most government regulations require that all of its minerals be removed. That includes the valuable mineral chromium, which is naturally found in foods that tend to be high in natural sugar. The chromium helps with the proper digestion and metabolism of naturally sweet foods. When it has been eliminated, we are prone to many of the health issues linked to white or refined sugar consumption, including weight gain.

While being overweight or obese can be a sign of a chromium deficiency, it is not the only one. Some other possible signs are cravings for sugary or starchy foods, diabetes or hypoglycemia (or chronically high or low blood sugar), difficulty tolerating alcohol or sugar, insulin resistance, syndrome X, metabolic syndrome, and high cholesterol or high triglyceride levels. But you can be deficient in chromium without experiencing any symptoms. Likewise, you can experience the weight-loss benefits of chromium supplementation even if you don't have a deficiency.

Chromium is also naturally found in many whole grains, romaine lettuce, onions, beans, legumes, and ripe tomatoes. Be sure to follow the guidelines for these foods as presented throughout *60 Seconds to Slim.*

How to Benefit

You can supplement with different types of chromium, but the one that has the greatest fat-burning effects is chromium glucose-tolerance factor, or chromium GTF. This is the form of chromium that is especially involved in balancing blood sugar levels, which likely accounts for its weight-loss benefits. Supplement with just 200 to 500 micrograms daily. According to research at the University of Texas, the benefits of chromium supplementation are superior when combined with conjugated linoleic acid (CLA).[5] Supplement with 2 to 3 grams (2,000 to 3,000 milligrams) of CLA daily for best results.

Many calcium supplements and antacids decrease the absorption of chromium, so it is best to take them separately from your chromium supplements. Conversely, aspirin is believed to increase chromium absorption, so if you are taking aspirin daily, you may need less chromium. It is important to follow dosage recommendations since chromium toxicity is possible, albeit rare.

If you are taking insulin or diabetes medications, consult your physician prior to taking chromium. He or she may need to adjust your medication because of chromium's ability to reduce high blood sugar levels.

Super Health Bonus

According to an interview with US Department of Agriculture research scientist Richard Anderson, PhD, "chromium is so helpful at controlling blood sugar, it could prevent diabetes in up to half of the at-risk people with higher-than-normal glucose levels."[6]

Chromium has also been shown to aid depression, according to Duke University researchers. Georgetown University Medical Center's Harry G. Preuss, MD, indicates that chromium supplementation also reduces the risk of heart attack by 41 percent.

60-Second Weight-Loss Tip #58:
Supplement with Fat to Lose Fat

Omega-3 fatty acids turn off your fat genes and increase the fat burned during exercise by 14 percent.[7]

Many people wrongly assume that to lose fat, you must reduce fat in your diet. And many health care practitioners continue to extoll this approach. While it is important to eliminate harmful fats from your diet to lose weight, it is also essential to add beneficial fats to propel weight loss. I'm referring to omega-3 fatty acids. Omega-3s turn off our fat-producing genes and turn on our fat-releasing genes, according to oil expert Udo Erasmus, PhD, in a recent interview.[8]

In a study, researchers found that consuming a diet high in omega-3–containing fish caused people's waistlines to shrink dramatically. Those who ate a high-fish diet saw their belly shrink between 4 and 6 inches, on average.[9]

Omega-3 fatty acids also lower levels of insulin to help control fluctuating blood sugar levels—a common problem linked to overweight or obesity. Fish also makes our bodies more receptive to the hormone leptin, which makes us feel full faster.

How to Benefit

Many food sources of omega-3 fatty acids, such as fish, flaxseeds, and walnuts, are discussed in more detail in Tip #21 on page 135. Alternatively, take approximately 2,000 milligrams daily of a fish oil supplement that contains both eicosapentaenoic acid (EPA) and docosahexaenoic acid (DHA).

Super Health Bonus

Omega-3 fatty acids not only help you lose belly fat and other excess weight, but they also help balance hormones and boost your immune system.

60-Second Weight-Loss Tip #59:
Inhale Vanilla to Stop Cravings

Inhaling the natural scent of vanilla can cause you to lose 5 pounds in 4 weeks without even trying.

There is a natural scent that, when inhaled, eliminates junk food cravings. What's more, the same scent, when inhaled regularly, causes people to lose an average of 5 pounds in 4 weeks without making any special effort, according to neurologist Alan R. Hirsch, MD, director of the Smell & Taste Treatment and Research Foundation in Chicago. The scent? Vanilla. The natural smell of vanilla stimulates the release of the brain chemical serotonin, a hormone that promotes feelings of satisfaction and happiness.[10]

Vanilla is the seedpod from a Central American orchid. Pure vanilla extract and vanilla essential oil are made by extracting the lovely aromatic scent. The former is an alcohol extract that is frequently used in baking. However, most of the "vanilla extracts" available for baking are synthetic and do not offer the therapeutic benefits of natural vanilla extract. Vanilla essential oil is made through the arduous task of extracting only the oil from the vanilla seedpods.

Dr. Hirsch indicates that the tendency to overeat is governed by the satiety center in the brain. He suggests that cravings can be eliminated simply by sniffing certain scents, especially when you have a tendency to overeat. And the smell of vanilla is one of the best scents to reduce cravings.[11]

Researchers at St. George's Hospital in London, England, conducted a test of a patch that adheres to the skin and releases the aroma of vanilla or other scents. They attempted to determine whether the patch, worn on the back of the hand, would reduce cravings for chocolate and sweet foods and beverages.

For the study, 200 overweight participants were divided into groups and received a vanilla patch, a lemon patch, a dummy patch, or no patch at all. After only 4 weeks, the weight lost in the other groups was a fraction of the weight lost by people wearing the vanilla patches.

According to Catherine Collins, the hospital's chief dietitian, who led the study, not only did the participants consume fewer sugary foods and beverages, but they also cut their chocolate consumption in half. What's more, the participants in the study lost an average of 4½ pounds simply from wearing the vanilla aroma patch.[12]

How to Benefit

Inhale only pure vanilla extract or vanilla essential oil. You can sniff it directly out of the bottle or place a few drops on a handkerchief and sniff it throughout the day. Ideally, smell the vanilla at least three times a day for 30 seconds each time; however, more often is fine too. The ideal time to inhale the wonderful scent of vanilla is when you are experiencing any cravings, since it can reduce your feelings of hunger. Be aware, however, that truly natural vanilla essential oil is usually thick. If it is thin, it has probably been diluted with a solvent and should be avoided. Don't worry if you can't find a good quality essential oil. You can get all the weight-loss benefits from a 100 percent pure vanilla extract, available in most health food stores and grocery stores.

Safety Consideration

You are probably familiar with vanilla-scented candles, vanilla fragrance oil used for potpourri and other household purposes, and vanilla perfume, all of which are typically made from synthetic vanilla and have no therapeutic purpose whatsoever. Instead, they may actually damage your body and cause it to hoard fat. Avoid these common items or you will be negating the benefits of the 60 Seconds to Slim program. Pure vanilla essential oil or vanilla extract will stain a handkerchief, so be sure to use one you don't mind staining.

Super Health Bonus

The fragrance of vanilla may help you cope with stress. Of study participants who smelled vanilla oil, 45 percent reported feeling relaxed while another 27 percent said they felt happy, according to research results published in the January 2005 supplement of *Chemical Senses*.[13]

Of 30 scents tested for their ability to increase penile bloodflow, vanilla was one to which older men reacted favorably, reported Dr. Hirsch of Chicago's Smell & Taste Treatment and Research Foundation.[14]

60-Second Weight-Loss Tip #60:
Take Bacteria to Transform Your Body's Inner Workings

Supplementing with probiotics transforms your inner terrain to that of a thin person.

As we discussed in 60-Second Weight-Loss Tip #32 on page 148, approximately half of your body's cells are actually bacteria and that an additional 100 trillion bacteria inhabit various parts of your body and play critical roles in your health. Don't let that scare you, however. You could not live without these microorganisms, most of which ensure a healthy flora balance in your body.

There are over 150 species of harmful yeasts known as candida, but the one that frequently becomes overgrown in our intestines is *Candida albicans*. The overgrowth of this yeast causes a common condition known as candidiasis. While it is rarely diagnosed by medical doctors, who often fail to recognize this commonplace and harmful condition, candidiasis can cause many negative health effects. Some of these symptoms are listed on page 218.

Probiotics are a group of microorganisms that play an essential role in ensuring the proper elimination of waste materials from the intestines, manufacturing important nutrients, controlling harmful bacteria and yeast populations like candida, and other necessary functions.

By eating foods high in probiotics or supplementing with these beneficial bacteria, you are helping to transform the terrain of your bowels to match that of thin people. This may not sound like a big deal, but it is. And here's why: Studies show that the levels of beneficial bacteria in a person's intestines can determine whether she will be fat or thin.

That's because the beneficial bacteria play a role in controlling harmful yeasts and bacteria in your body, as well as metabolizing food, extracting the nutrients your body needs, and even controlling appetite. Probiotics play a huge role in your weight and health. Many different types of probiotics are beneficial to your weight-loss efforts, but the *Lactobacillus* strains are particularly linked to appetite control by helping to maintain stable blood sugar levels, which translates into fewer cravings for unhealthful foods, fewer fat storage hormones, and less intense hunger.

Probiotics also work by keeping the balance between different types of bacteria in your intestines. Exciting research published in the journal *Internal and Emergency Medicine* indicates that probiotics may help balance the intestinal bacterial flora in humans, with promising preliminary results in the prevention and treatment of obesity and metabolic disorders.[15]

How can you tell if you are suffering from candidiasis? Here are some of the symptoms.

- Acne
- Bloating
- Bruising easily
- Cold sores, canker sores, or herpes simplex
- Constipation
- Diarrhea
- Eczema or psoriasis
- Heart disease
- Hemorrhoids
- High cholesterol
- Indigestion
- Intestinal gas
- Irritable bowel syndrome
- Nosebleeds
- Urinary tract infections (also bladder or kidney infections, also called cystitis)
- Yeast infections or candida overgrowth

How to Benefit

Many foods contain probiotics, including fermented soy foods like miso and tempeh, naturally fermented sauerkraut, kimchi, and other naturally pickled foods (those pickled in vinegar do not have the same benefits). Keep in mind that I am referring to unsweetened, preservative- and artificial color–free foods best found in a natural foods store. Also, many books and health experts tell people that tofu is a fermented food, but in most cases, it is not. Having visited tofu manufacturing plants, I can say with confidence that tofu is not a fermented food. Or you can make your own naturally fermented foods. It is much easier than you might think. I have included a recipe for homemade probiotic-rich dairy-free soft "Cheese" at the back of this book (see page 250). If you are purchasing foods that contain probiotics, be sure that they are labeled as containing "live, active cultures," since most foods have been processed at temperatures that destroy the beneficial bacteria.

Also, be aware that many foods claim to contain *prebiotics,* which is not the same thing as probiotics. Prebiotics are sugars that help to feed probiotic cultures. There is a lot of hype around prebiotic foods, most of which is ill deserved.

You may be wondering why, if probiotic bacteria normally reside in your intestine, you should supplement them. Over time, probiotics can become depleted or destroyed by harmful microbes, excess sugar consumption, antibiotic use, and many other factors. It is important to replenish your body's stores with a probiotic supplement.

Choose a supplement that contains *Lactobacillus acidophilus* (also called *L. acidophilus*), *L. bifidus, Bacillus subtilis, L. casei, L. bulgaris, L. plantarum, L. paracasei, L. rhamnosus, L. salivarius, L. longum, L. lactis, L. F19,* and *Bifidobacterium bifidum.* Don't worry if you can't find one that contains all of these bacterial strains. Simply choose the most comprehensive one you can find.

Take two capsules of probiotics daily on an empty stomach. I usually recommend taking them first thing in the morning or in the evening, before bed. If you take them in the morning, wait at least 20 minutes before eating. I usually take probiotics with a large glass of water with fresh lemon juice upon awakening, shower, and then eat breakfast. This is an easy routine to get into and helps to put some time between your probiotics and breakfast.

Supplementing with probiotics or eating probiotic-rich food may not be sufficient if you have yeast overgrowth in your intestines. You'll still need to follow a low-sugar, low-carb program like the one outlined in *60 Seconds to Slim.* That's because harmful yeasts feed on sugars, and most carbs break down into sugars. Nonstarchy vegetables are the exception. While they are carbohydrates, they usually are quite low in natural sugars. While some complex carbohydrates such as beans and some whole grains break down into sugars, when eaten in small amounts, they usually do so at a slow rate that will not increase yeast populations. Also, check out Tip #62 on page 223 for another natural remedy that kills candida.

Super Health Bonus

Many great health bonuses are linked to probiotic supplementation. Here are some of the main benefits. After reading this list, I'm sure you'll be as convinced as I am that probiotic supplementation is one of the best things you can do for your body.

BENEFITS OF PROBIOTICS

- Help digest food and ensure that the nutrients are synthesized and absorbed by the body
- Help to ensure that toxins are not absorbed into the blood while keeping harmful bacteria in check, thereby aiding gut and immune system health
- Improve nasal and sinus symptoms linked to allergies, according to research by scientists at the Osaka University School of Medicine[16]
- Reduce inflammatory response linked to diabetes, heart disease, and other chronic illnesses, according to research published in the journal *Gut Microbes*[17]
- May reduce likelihood of developing colitis, according to research at the University of British Columbia, Canada[18]
- May aid in the treatment and management of celiac disease, according to research published in the *Scandinavian Journal of Immunology*[19]
- Improve the symptoms of rheumatoid arthritis, according to scientists at the University of Western Ontario, Canada[20]
- Improve nutritional quality in the breast milk of women who supplement their diet with *Lactobacillus rhamnosus* and *Bifidobacterium lactis,* according to scientists at the University of Turku, Finland[21]
- Show antiviral activity against the herpes simplex type 2 virus, according to scientists at Sapienza University, Italy[22]

- Can prevent or shorten the duration of a cold by competing with viruses[23]

- Lower negative immune system compounds called cytokines, not only in the gut, but also throughout the bloodstream (cytokines are linked to anxiety and symptoms of depression, among other symptoms in healthy adults)[24]

- Can lower oxidative stress in the body; according to a study by Swedish researchers in the *American Journal of Clinical Nutrition,* oral administration of a strain of probiotics called *Lactobacillus plantarum* resulted in a 37 percent reduction in chemicals that mark oxidative stress in the body and that are elevated in many brain and neurological diseases[25]

- Can inhibit the growth of *Helicobacter pylori*—the bacteria that has been linked to stomach ulcers[26]

- May help heal respiratory infections according to research published in the *British Journal of Nutrition*[27]

60-Second Weight-Loss Tip #61:
Supplement with Calcium to Neutralize Acid

Calcium is a superalkaline mineral that neutralizes acid to boost your weight loss.

You learned earlier that one of your body's coping methods for neutralizing acidity is to withdraw calcium from your bones. Calcium is an alkalizing mineral that is a natural antacid. Like a bank account from which regular withdrawals are made, your bones can become vulnerable to excessive losses. Yet calcium is a beneficial weight-loss mineral, probably for a multitude of reasons, but definitely for its ability to help your body to become more alkaline.

Jennifer Leigh Rosenblum, MD, and associates at the Massachusetts General Hospital Weight Center and Gastrointestinal Unit in Boston assessed several studies to determine the effect of calcium and vitamin D supplementation on weight. They found a highly significant decrease in abdominal fat in overweight and obese individuals.[28]

Another meta-analysis of calcium supplementation for weight loss was jointly conducted by the University of Exeter and the Peninsula College of Medicine and Dentistry in the United Kingdom. The scientists published their results in the journal *Nutrition Review*. They found that supplementation with calcium resulted in statistically significant weight loss in overweight and obese individuals.[29]

How to Benefit

To help restore the amount of calcium in your body, you can supplement with this critical mineral. Everyone's needs are different, but they usually range from 800 to 1,500 milligrams daily. The more alkaline your diet, the lower your needs will likely be, but a menopausal or postmenopausal woman may still require 1,500 milligrams daily. Not all calcium supplements are created equal, however, and some can even be contaminated with lead. Choose calcium citrate, as it is a highly absorbable form. Also, make sure the brand you choose has third-party, independent laboratory tests that show low parts per million of the heavy metal lead. Ideally, take vitamin D and magnesium along with your calcium.

Safety Consideration

In the same way that the bones act as a reserve for alkaline calcium, your muscles are reservoirs for the mineral magnesium, which is also alkaline. Most nutrition experts estimate that 80 percent of people are deficient in this important mineral. For best results, it is best to take calcium and magnesium together. Otherwise a deficiency can develop in the mineral that is not supplemented. Most people take between 400 and 800 milligrams of magnesium daily.

Super Health Bonus

Not only will you build stronger bones and teeth, but if you supplement with magnesium along with calcium, you may reduce muscle tension, pain, and headaches too. That's because magnesium is the muscle relaxant of natural medicine.

60-Second Weight-Loss Tip #62:
Take Grape Seed Extract to Stop Belly Fat Formation

Grape seed extract is proven to stop the formation of belly fat in its tracks.

According to a study published in the journal *Molecular Nutrition and Food Research,* animals given grape seed extract built up less abdominal fat than animals not given the supplement. Researchers found that the animals given grape seed extract had a whopping 61 percent increase in adiponectin, a hormone that speeds the conversion of fat and triglycerides into energy.[30]

For those people wondering whether they can glean these weight-loss benefits from drinking wine, sorry, the answer is definitely no.

How to Benefit

While this study was done on animals, the scientists who conducted it believe its findings will translate to humans as well. It's easy to benefit from the research. Simply take a supplement of 200 milligrams of grape seed extract daily to help your body convert fat stores into energy and to slow the accumulation of more belly fat.

You can also blend organic grapes that contain seeds with some water in a blender for a delicious juice. But this drink is best reserved for after you've lost the weight you want to lose since it is high in natural sugars.

Safety Consideration

Choose a high-quality grape seed extract supplement. Inferior ones are solvent extracted and may contain some residue of the chemical solvent used to extract the therapeutic benefits from grape seeds. Unfortunately, this is difficult to discern from the bottle. Speak to your local health food store owner or contact the manufacturer directly to determine whether solvents are used. I use Pranarom brand, but there are other excellent ones too.

Super Health Benefit

Grape seed extract is a potent and proven antibacterial, antifungal, antiviral, and antiparasitic agent. In other words, it kills nasty critters linked to all sorts of illnesses, from candida overgrowth to viral diseases. So while you're benefiting from its weight-loss properties, you'll also be killing any unwanted infections you might have.

60-Second Weight-Loss Tip #63:
Take Carnitine to Burn Fat Fast

Carnitine is a powerful nutrient that transports fat to your cells' incinerators to be burned as fuel.

Your body is the ultimate alchemist. With the help of a powerful nutrient, it can burn fat to create energy. I know it sounds like something out of a science fiction movie, but extensive research shows that this miracle nutrient actually burns fat while giving people more energy.

Exciting new research keeps pouring in about the powerful fat-blasting abilities of the vitamin-like nutrient carnitine. Most people get only about 50 milligrams of carnitine in their daily diet, but this is not enough for optimal health and it is insufficient to cause weight loss. The body can make this important nutrient from other nutrients we consume, such as lysine, methionine, vitamin C, iron, niacin, and vitamin B_6, so it's technically not an essential nutrient; however, a deficiency in any of these nutrients can cause a deficiency in carnitine, which may explain why carnitine deficiency is quite common. Some of the symptoms of a carnitine deficiency include overweight, fatigue, heart problems, and high levels of triglycerides.

In a recent study, participants were divided into two groups: those who ate a healthy diet and exercised moderately and those who ate healthy, exercised moderately, and supplemented with 2 grams of carnitine daily. The results were astounding. Those who supplemented with carnitine lost an average of 11 pounds, while the former group lost only 1 pound in 12 weeks.[31]

According to carnitine expert and author of *The Carnitine Miracle* Robert Crayhon, MS, the reason carnitine is so effective for weight loss is "because carnitine is the forklift that takes fat to the incinerators in our cells called mitochondria. Unless fat makes it into the mitochondria, you can't burn it off. . . . Once fat is inside the mitochondria fat is magically transformed into energy."[32]

Carnitine also powers up your endurance, so you'll start to notice that you can walk longer or work out longer without getting as tired. Research even shows that people who work out only once or twice a week start to perform as though they had greater levels of conditioning.[33]

How to Benefit

You'll need to supplement with at least 500 milligrams to feel a difference and to reap the fat-burning benefits. Some people don't notice the difference until they take 2,000 to 3,000 milligrams daily. Choose carnitine tartrate for the best results, since it is the purest and most effective form of the nutrient. It's best taken early in the day on an empty stomach, ideally before breakfast.

Safety Consideration

Avoid taking carnitine after 3 p.m. since it may give you more energy than you'd like when you're ready to sleep.

Super Health Bonus

Carnitine also boosts heart health. Two-thirds of the energy needed to fuel the heart is derived from burning fat. Because carnitine helps us to burn fat more efficiently, it helps the heart to get sufficient energy for proper functioning. This is particularly true for people suffering from congestive heart failure. Carnitine also helps to clear the arteries, lower high triglycerides, and raise good HDL cholesterol, known for its heart protective properties. That's great news for anyone with heart disease, high blood pressure, or another heart condition.

60-Second Weight-Loss Tip #64:
Mop Up Free Radicals with Lipoic Acid

Lipoic acid is a powerful antioxidant that mops up free radicals linked to inflammation, weight gain, and disease.

Lipoic acid is a powerful antioxidant that has the ability to clear out free radicals linked to inflammation, weight gain, aging, and disease. Additionally, within cells, it has the ability to increase the production of leptin, which appears to stifle the production of the chemical ghrelin, linked to increased appetite. In other words, lipoic acid can help turn off hunger pangs. Overweight women taking lipoic acid in scientific studies were found to have lost 5 percent of their body weight within 6 months.[34]

Lipoic acid has also been shown to power up the energy centers of the cells, called mitochondria, helping them to work more effectively. That means improved fat burning and increased energy for you! Researchers at the University of California, Berkeley, found that lipoic acid had the ability to double energy levels in their subjects.

How to Benefit

Lipoic acid is found in plentiful amounts in dark leafy greens, including kale, Swiss chard, collard greens, and spinach. Eat more of these vegetables. But to really obtain the benefits found in the study, you'll need more lipoic acid than you can obtain normally through diet. So supplement with 100 to 300 milligrams of lipoic acid—or alpha lipoic acid, as it is also called.

Super Health Bonus

You'll turn back the clock on wrinkling and many other age-related conditions while improving your energy levels. New research shows that lipoic acid protects the eyes against damage linked to free radicals and aging.[35] It also helped reverse memory loss linked to age-related brain decline.[36] A supplement that reverses the effects of aging, causes weight loss, and boosts energy? No, this isn't a fairy tale. This is nutritional science at its finest.

60-Second Weight-Loss Tip #65:
Detoxify More Fat with Natural Herbs

Milk thistle, dandelion, globe artichoke, and turmeric boost your liver's ability to break down harmful fats, excessive hormones, and toxins linked to weight gain.

MILK THISTLE (*SILYBUM MARIANUM*)

If you've ever walked barefoot in the grass and stepped on a prickly weed, you're already familiar with one herb that detoxifies harmful toxins, fats, and hormones linked to weight gain. You may have cursed it rather than sung its praises. Called milk thistle, or *Silybum marianum,* this prickly herb contains a powerful phytonutrient called silymarin in its seeds.

Silymarin protects the liver by inhibiting damaging substances that cause liver cell damage. This compound also stimulates liver cell regeneration to help the liver rebuild after it has been damaged. And it helps to prevent the depletion of the nutrient glutathione—one of the most critical nutrients for liver detoxification. Silymarin also has anti-inflammatory and antioxidant abilities and may be helpful in reducing the growth of cancer cells.[37] It is traditionally used by natural health practitioners to support the detoxification of the liver and to strengthen this organ.

But milk thistle is not the only herb that boosts liver function. There are many. If you can't locate milk thistle, you can choose from some of my other favorite herbal liver boosters.

DANDELION ROOT (*TARAXACUM OFFICINALE*)

Nature grows a liver-cleansing pharmacy every spring, in the form of the dreaded weed that most people curse as it pokes its yellow-flowered head through the green of their lawn. Dandelion is one of Mother Nature's finest liver herbs. The *Australian Journal of Medical Herbalism* cited two studies that showed the liver-regenerative properties of dandelion in cases of jaundice, liver swelling, hepatitis, and indigestion.

GLOBE ARTICHOKE (*CYNARA SCOLYMUS*)

Globe artichoke contains compounds called caffeoylquinic acids that have demonstrated powerful liver-regenerating effects similar to those of milk thistle.

TURMERIC (*CURCUMA LONGA*)

A spice commonly used in Indian curries, turmeric helps regenerate liver cells and cleanse the liver of toxins. Turmeric also increases the production of bile to help expel toxins and may help reduce liver inflammation. In studies turmeric has also been shown to increase levels of two liver-supporting enzymes that promote phase II liver detoxification reactions.

How to Benefit

Silymarin in **milk thistle** seeds is not water soluble, so it does not extract well into tea. Instead, take a standardized extract containing about 140 milligrams of silymarin for liver cleansing and protection.

If you choose to incorporate **dandelion root** into your liver-cleansing efforts, take 500 to 2,000 milligrams daily in capsules. Alternatively, you can combine 2 teaspoons of powdered dandelion root with 1 cup of water. Bring to a boil and simmer for 15 minutes. Drink 1 cup, three times daily.

Globe artichoke is usually found in capsule form. Doses range from 300 to 500 milligrams daily.

Turmeric comes in capsules and tablets, sometimes labeled "curcumin," which is its key ingredient. The dose will be higher if you are taking turmeric than if you take it's active ingredient curcumin. Mix 1 teaspoon turmeric in a glass of water and drink 3 to 4 glasses daily. Or, take 400 milligrams of curcumin three times daily for best results. You can also add ground turmeric to soups, stews, and curries.

Super Health Bonus

Regardless of which herb you choose to boost your liver function, you'll be reducing your cancer risk. However, if you choose turmeric or curcumin, you'll also notice its impressive ability to quell pain and inflammation. Expect fewer joint and muscle aches, headaches, and other types of pain.

60-Second SUCCESS STORY

Gloria Yackimec

Age: **56**
Location: **Alberta, Canada**
Occupation: **Licensed practical nurse working in an emergency/OR department**

Total Weight Lost:
8 pounds

Total Inches Lost:
7

> "Lemon water, green tea, greens, and pH drops have become staples in my daily diet."

How I Got Here:

Gloria's story is a familiar one: An injury makes it difficult to exercise and easy to gain weight. She says, "Prior to the onset of this program, I was feeling somewhat tired and sluggish while experiencing pain and inflammation from a rotator cuff injury." Additionally, she says, "Being a shift worker can have a tendency of throwing off any regular routines such as good eating and exercising schedules."

Gloria adds, "My personal goals were to increase my energy levels and general well-being while losing a few pounds. The program looked inviting and it was a wonderful opportunity to be mentored by Dr. Schoffro Cook on how to eat healthy while losing a few pounds. She has many good suggestions as well as recipes for achieving weight-loss goals."

(continued)

Progress Report:

"Although exercise has routinely been a part of my life, I noticed a significant surge in energy—mentally, physically, and emotionally—shortly after switching to a more alkaline diet," Gloria says. "Lemon water, green tea, greens, and pH drops have become staples in my daily diet. I especially enjoy trying new recipes that are predominately alkaline in a world of prepared, processed, acidic foods." Gloria decided to stay on the program for 6 weeks total. She says, "I found it an uplifting, rewarding experience and am continuing to use some of the tips, knowing that I can restart the whole program at any time."

Beyond:

Gloria lost 8 pounds and 7 inches. She says, "I am happy with my results. I am one size smaller and my clothes fit better. [The program] gave me more insight as to how detrimental a consistent high-acidic diet can be to my health, as 1 week into the program there was a notable decrease of pain to my arm."

Going forward, Gloria states: "I will be more conscientious about balancing my alkaline and acidic food choices to promote a healthier lifestyle."

PART 3

RECIPES

Chapter 7

Recipes

Here are some of my favorite recipes. While they are not all alkalizing (some are Wise Acid choices), they are designed to fit into the 60 Seconds to Slim program, showing you all the ways you can alkalize your body without sacrificing the delicious foods you are accustomed to. I was sure to include breakfast options, since this is an area where people sometimes have a hard time finding alkaline choices, as well as options for lunch, dinner, snacks, and desserts.

Many of these mouthwatering recipes were submitted by my friends and colleagues: Cobi Slater, PhD, DNM, CHT, RNCP, ROHP, from Maple Ridge, British Columbia—creator of Essential Health Natural Wellness Clinic and EatCleanMenus.com; Angela Grow, recipe developer and wellness coach from Salmon Creek, Washington, who helped her husband, Bobby, overcome cancer with an alkaline diet; and Denise Passerello, MS, CPT, CNC, a nutritionist and creator of the excellent Web site Fresh-Fitness.com.

Bon appétit!

Breakfasts

Beverages

Appetizers, Dips, and Spreads

Soups

Salads and Salad Dressings

Entrées

Side Dishes

Desserts

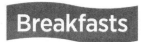
Breakfasts

Hot Breakfast Cereal

Most grains are acid forming and can make weight loss a struggle. However, quinoa (pronounced KEEN-wah*), an ancient seed, makes a delicious and nutritious breakfast. It takes only 15 minutes to cook and is alkalizing. For those mornings when you are rushed, cook the quinoa in advance; then gently reheat and add almond milk and cinnamon for a quick, easy, and satisfying breakfast.*

1   **cup golden quinoa**

1½   **cups water**

1   **cup unsweetened almond milk**

1   **teaspoon ground cinnamon**

In a small saucepan, place the quinoa and water. Cover. Bring to a boil, then reduce the heat and simmer for 15 minutes or until the water has been absorbed. Remove from the heat. Place in bowls. Stir in the almond milk and cinnamon.

MAKES 4 SERVINGS

Per serving: 182 calories, 6 g protein, 32 g carbohydrates, 4 g total fat, 0 g saturated fat, 4 g fiber, 59 mg sodium

Lots 'o Seeds Whole Grain Cereal

When my friend Angela Grow first shared this recipe, I had to try it immediately. From the ingredient list I could tell it was a powerhouse of nutrition (rich in protein, fiber, essential fats, vitamins, minerals, and phytonutrients). After trying it, I was pleased to note that it is as good tasting as it is good for you. Angela helped her husband, Bobby Grow, overcome cancer using an alkaline diet.

4	cups gluten-free oats
¼	cup ground flaxseeds
¼	cup pumpkin seeds
¼	cup sunflower seeds
1	teaspoon ground cinnamon
½	cup raisins or dried cranberries (optional, as it does add sugar; be sure to choose unsulphured fruit that's not coated in oil, which is available at most health food stores)

In a large bowl, combine the oats, flaxseeds, pumpkin seeds, sunflower seeds, cinnamon, and raisins or cranberries, if using. Serve with almond or coconut milk for a filling and hearty breakfast cereal, or store for later as a trail mix–type snack.

MAKES 4 SERVINGS

Per serving: 464 calories, 20 g protein, 60 g carbohydrates, 16 g total fat, 2.5 g saturated fat, 11 g fiber, 2 mg sodium

Basic Spelt Muffins

My friend Angela Grow shared this wonderful muffin recipe with me.
Her kids love them. Once you taste them, you'll understand why.

2	cups spelt flour
½	cup palm sugar or coconut sap
2½	teaspoons aluminum-free baking powder
½	teaspoon sea salt
½	cup coconut oil
1	egg or 1 tablespoon ground flaxseeds combined with 3 tablespoons water
1	cup unsweetened almond milk
1	cup fruit, nuts, and/or seeds (cranberries, blueberries, chopped apples, walnuts, almonds, or your choice)

Preheat the oven to 400°F. Grease a 12-cup muffin tin with coconut oil.

In a large mixing bowl, combine the flour, palm sugar or coconut sap, baking powder, and salt. In a saucepan over low heat, warm the oil until it melts but is not hot.

In a separate bowl, combine the melted oil, egg or flaxseed mixture, and almond milk. Add the egg mixture to the flour mixture, being careful not to overmix. Gently fold in your choice of fruit, nuts, and/or seeds. Pour the batter into the muffin tin. Bake for 15 minutes or until a wooden pick inserted in the center of a muffin comes out clean. Remove from the oven and let cool in the tin for a few minutes, then remove to a cooling rack. The muffins will keep in an airtight container for 2 days.

MAKES 12

Variation: You may decrease the palm sugar or coconut sap to ¼ cup and add ½ teaspoon of liquid stevia to reduce the amount of sugar in each muffin.

Per muffin: 194 calories, 3 g protein, 20 g carbohydrates, 11 g total fat, 8.5 g saturated fat, 3 g fiber, 212 mg sodium

Maple-Fennel Sausage

Okay, I can probably guess what you're thinking. What's a recipe for sausage doing in a healthy weight-loss book like this? But bear with me. This delicious and lean turkey sausage is a great Wise Acid addition to the largely alkaline 60 Seconds to Slim program. I make enough to have leftovers to freeze, and then I pan-fry a couple of patties whenever I want them. The fenugreek seeds impart the maple flavor without adding any sugar. Actually, fenugreek is excellent to help regulate blood sugar and, as you learned earlier, blood sugar balance is essential to weight loss. The fennel seeds aid digestion and add a delicious flavor.

1	large onion, chopped + ½ onion
2	large carrots, finely chopped
2	ribs celery, finely chopped
1	tablespoon coconut oil
1	clove garlic
1	tablespoon fennel seeds
2	teaspoons fenugreek seeds or ground fenugreek
1	teaspoon freshly ground black peppercorns
1	teaspoon dried basil
1	teaspoon Himalayan crystal salt or Celtic sea salt
½	teaspoon dried thyme
½	cup whole grain flour, preferably gluten free
4	pounds 93% lean, organic ground turkey
2	large organic eggs

Preheat the oven to 350°F.

In a skillet over low to medium heat, cook the chopped onion, carrots, and celery in the oil, stirring frequently, until lightly browned. Be sure not to let the oil smoke. Let cool.

In a food processor, finely chop the remaining ½ onion and the garlic. Add the cooked vegetables and pulse until coarsely chopped.

In a large bowl, place the vegetable mixture and fennel seeds, fenugreek, peppercorns, basil, salt, thyme, and flour. Combine until thoroughly mixed. Add the turkey and eggs and mix together until the vegetables and seasonings are evenly distributed.

Cut a sheet of unbleached parchment paper into 2 pieces of approximately 1-foot lengths. Place half of the ground turkey mixture in the center of each parchment piece and shape into 2 large logs. Tightly wrap the parchment around each log and place both logs together in a baking pan.

Bake for 1 hour. Cool, then refrigerate for at least 1 hour. Remove the parchment from the turkey logs and slice into ½" disks. To freeze the sausage, lay the disks on a baking sheet and place it in the freezer. Once the sausage patties are frozen, place them in freezer bags and keep frozen until needed.

To serve, pan-fry sausage patties until lightly browned on both sides.

MAKES 20

Per patty: 154 calories, 19 g protein, 5 g carbohydrates, 7 g total fat, 2.5 g saturated fat, 1 g fiber, 119 mg sodium

Gluten-Free Pancakes

If you're looking for a delicious, hearty start in the morning that will keep you going throughout the day, try these pancakes. They're also packed with alkaline- and calcium-rich almonds and almond milk to aid fat burning. Just go easy on the maple syrup (fresh fruit is preferable as a topping), and definitely stay clear of "pancake syrup" or "maple-like" syrups. They are usually just high fructose corn syrup and synthetic maple flavors disguised as the real thing.

1	**cup almond flour**
½	**cup tapioca flour**
1	**teaspoon baking soda**
2	**teaspoons palm sugar or coconut sap**
1	**egg**
1½	**cups almond milk or coconut milk**
½	**teaspoon coconut oil**

In a large mixing bowl, combine the flours, baking soda, and palm sugar or coconut sap. In a separate bowl, whisk together the egg and almond milk or coconut milk. Gradually pour the egg mixture into the flour mixture, whisking constantly until just mixed. In a medium to large skillet over low to medium heat, heat the oil. When the pan is hot and evenly greased, scoop some batter into the pan with a large ladle. Cook until lightly golden on the bottom or until the bubbles pop and the pancake is slightly dry on top. Flip. Cook for 30 seconds to 1 minute. Continue in the same way until all the batter is used.

MAKES 6

Per pancake: 176 calories, 5 g protein, 16 g carbohydrates, 11 g total fat, 1 g saturated fat, 2 g fiber, 266 mg sodium

Coconut Waffles

Okay, waffles are not exactly a weight-loss food, but these can be eaten on occasion (no more than 2 per week) as a treat. They are loaded with medium-chain triglycerides, which help speed up the thyroid. The shredded coconut helps boost the fiber content as well. I love them topped with raspberries or blueberries.

5	cups gluten-free or spelt flour (such as Bob's Red Mill gluten-free all-purpose blend)
1	cup shredded unsweetened coconut
2	teaspoons baking soda
1	teaspoon ground cinnamon
1	tablespoon palm sugar or coconut sap
5	cups coconut milk
2	eggs
2	tablespoons coconut oil

In a large mixing bowl, combine the flour, coconut, baking soda, cinnamon, and palm sugar or coconut sap. In a separate bowl, combine the coconut milk, eggs, and oil, whisking until blended. Then pour the egg mixture into the flour mixture and stir just until blended. Pour into a waffle maker and cook according to the manufacturer's instructions. Enjoy topped with berries for a delicious treat. Alternatively, freeze on a parchment-lined baking sheet and, once frozen, place in a sealed freezer bag for later use.

MAKES 24

Per waffle: 214 calories, 4 g protein, 22 g carbohydrates, 14 g total fat, 11 g saturated fat, 3 g fiber, 127 mg sodium

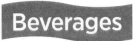
Beverages

Minty Melon Refresher

This icy drink is perfect on a hot summer day when you need refreshment. It's cooling, calming, and oh so delicious. The sweet watermelon with the mint leaves is a fantastic combination.

2	cups seeded and coarsely chopped watermelon
10	ice cubes
4	mint leaves

In a blender, combine the watermelon, ice cubes, and mint. Blend until smooth. Serve immediately.

MAKES 1 SERVING

Per serving: 80 calories, 1 g protein, 21 g carbohydrates, 0 g total fat, 0 g saturated fat, 1 g fiber, 6 mg sodium

Super Fat-Busting Green Tea Lemonade

Now you can reap all the fat-busting benefits of green tea lemonade without the excessive amount of calories. This pH-neutral tea will fire up your metabolism—and it even tastes sweet, thanks to stevia.

1	quart or liter pure alkaline water
6	green tea bags
½	cup fresh lemon juice
10–20	drops liquid stevia, or to taste
2	cups ice, or as needed
1	sprig fresh mint (optional)

In a kettle, bring the water to a boil. Add the tea bags and let them steep for 5 to 10 minutes. In a bowl, add the lemon juice and the stevia. Once the tea has finished steeping, add the ice and allow the tea to cool before pouring into a pitcher and adding the lemon juice and stevia mixture (putting it in the refrigerator will help speed cooling). Stir until mixed and enjoy served over additional ice. Garnish with a sprig of mint, if desired.

MAKES 2 SERVINGS

Per serving: 15 calories, 1 g protein, 5 g carbohydrates, 0 g total fat, 0 g saturated fat, 1 g fiber, 26 mg sodium

Alkalizing Almond Milk

While you can buy unsweetened almond milk if you prefer, it is easy to make your own. Add it to cooked quinoa for a delicious hot breakfast cereal, use it as a base for smoothies or as a substitute for milk in baked goods, or enjoy it on its own, chilled, with a dash of vanilla extract, as a refreshing alkaline beverage.

2	cups purified water
½	cup almonds
6–10	drops liquid stevia, or to taste

In a blender, combine the water, almonds, and stevia. Blend until smooth. Strain if you plan to use the almond milk for baking.

MAKES 2 SERVINGS

VARIATION:

Add 1 teaspoon pure vanilla extract or vanilla powder for a delicious vanilla almond milk.

Per serving: 206 calories, 8 g protein, 8 g carbohydrates, 18 g total fat, 1.5 g saturated fat, 4 g fiber, 1 mg sodium

Appetizers, Dips, and Spreads

Buckwheat Flatbread

These dense flatbreads are delicious and versatile and make great plat-forms for savory or sweet snacks. They are perfect for dipping into hummus or guacamole or eating as an occasional treat with berries. You can make them silver-dollar size for appetizers, canapés, or snacks. Or make them larger as a side dish for your meal. They're extremely satisfying, thanks to their plentiful fiber.

2	cups buckwheat flour
1	teaspoon baking soda
2½	cups unsweetened almond milk
2	organic eggs
½	teaspoon extra virgin coconut oil

In a large mixing bowl, combine the flour and baking soda. In a separate bowl, whisk together the almond milk and eggs. Add the egg mixture to the flour mixture and whisk together until just mixed. In a large skillet over medium heat, heat the oil. Using a medium ladle, drop the batter onto the skillet and cook until no bubbles remain on the surface. Flip and cook for another 30 seconds to 1 minute. Repeat until all the batter is used.

MAKES 6

Per flatbread: 177 calories, 8 g protein, 29 g carbohydrates, 4 g total fat, 1 g saturated fat, 6 g fiber, 306 mg sodium

Quinoa Flatbread

These versatile flatbreads are made like crepes. I stuff them with cooked quinoa, curry spices, chickpeas, onions, and tomatoes and grill them on a panini press for a healthy and delicious pocket-type sandwich. Alternatively, I stuff them with hummus, sprouts, lettuce, and grated carrot for a salad on the go. They're best made with a healthy nonstick pan like Paderno's Eco Pans.

2	cups tapioca flour
1	cup quinoa flour
1	cup ground almonds
1½	teaspoons baking soda
3	cups almond milk
2	eggs
½	teaspoon coconut oil

In a large bowl, combine the flours, almonds, and baking soda. Add the almond milk and eggs. Whisk everything together. In a skillet over low to medium heat, heat the oil. When it is hot enough to cause a single drop of batter to sizzle but not so hot that the oil smokes, spoon the batter into the skillet and move it in circles to make thin, crepelike flatbreads. Once the surface no longer has bubbles and looks heated through (after 1 minute), flip and cook for an additional 30 seconds. Continue until you've used up all the batter, adding more oil to the skillet as necessary.

MAKES 8

Per flatbread: 271 calories, 6 g protein, 42 g carbohydrates, 9 g total fat, 1 g saturated fat, 4 g fiber, 314 mg sodium

Alkalizing Butter Substitute

This rich and delicious butter substitute is a fat-busting powerhouse. It contains omega-3 fatty acids that burn fat and medium-chain triglycerides that reset the body's metabolism gland—the thyroid. It's best added to foods after they've been cooked, as the delicate omega-3 fatty acids are damaged when heated during cooking. Enjoy on steamed or sautéed vegetables, on a piece of warm bread, or atop a steaming bowl of quinoa or other alkaline grain.

¾   **cup extra virgin coconut oil**

¾   **cup cold-pressed flax oil**

In a small saucepan over low heat, liquefy the coconut oil. Remove the pan from the heat immediately after all the solids have liquefied. Add the flax oil and stir until well mixed. Pour into a glass container with a lid and refrigerate until firm. Store in the refrigerator for up to 6 months.

MAKES 24 SERVINGS (1 TABLESPOON PER SERVING)

Per serving: 125 calories, 0 g protein, 0 g carbohydrates, 14 g total fat, 7 g saturated fat, 0 g fiber, 0 mg sodium

Dairy-Free Soft "Cheese"

This "cheese" is so delicious no one will know it's a healthy, dairy-free option. It offers all the benefits of yogurt (including weight loss) without the lymphatic-system-clogging dairy. Plus, it helps to balance your bowel flora. While it requires half a day for fermentation, it takes only about 5 to 10 minutes of preparation time in the kitchen.

2	cups raw, unsalted cashews, soaked overnight or for 10–12 hours
1	teaspoon probiotic powder or 2 probiotic capsules, opened (available in most health food stores; sometimes called *L. acidophilus* or *flora*), dissolved in 1 cup pure water
1	teaspoon Celtic sea salt or Himalayan crystal salt, or to taste
1–2	teaspoons onion powder
¼	teaspoon ground nutmeg

In a blender or food processor, combine the cashews and the probiotic powder and water mixture. Blend until smooth. Place in a glass bowl, cover with a clean cloth, and let rest for 10 to 14 hours to ferment. Then stir in the salt, onion powder, and nutmeg until well mixed. Form the cheese into a ball or press it into a spring-form pan. Serve with crackers, pitas, or vegetable crudités.

MAKES APPROXIMATELY 2 CUPS OF CHEESE, OR 12 SERVINGS

VARIATIONS:

- Add a teaspoon or two of herbs, such as herbes de Provence, to flavor the cheese once it has fermented or to coat the outside of a cheese ball.
- Serve the cheese coated with ground or chopped nuts, such as hazelnuts.
- Serve the cheese drizzled with a balsamic vinegar reduction.

Per serving: 105 calories, 3 g protein, 6 g carbohydrates, 8 g total fat, 1.5 g saturated fat, 1 g fiber, 200 mg sodium

Stedda Feta

This quinoa tastes like cheese and makes a great high-protein, high-fiber option to use on salads or whenever you just crave cheese. It is also great on crackers or flatbreads. I enjoy eating it on its own sometimes as a side dish or scooped up with ribs of celery. Quinoa and lemon juice are both alkalizing foods.

1	cup quinoa
1¾	cups water or amount shown in quinoa package directions
½	teaspoon unrefined sea salt
2	tablespoons fresh lemon juice

In a small pot, combine the quinoa and water. Bring to a boil and then simmer for 15 to 20 minutes, or according to package directions. Cool, then add the salt and lemon juice. Toss until mixed. Let marinate for at least 10 minutes.

MAKES 6 SERVINGS

Per serving: 106 calories, 4 g protein, 19 g carbohydrates, 2 g total fat, 0.5 g saturated fat, 2 g fiber, 201 mg sodium

Hummus

Hummus is a delicious Middle Eastern and Mediterranean dip that is as delicious as it is versatile. Most store-bought brands contain harmful preservatives or acid-forming ingredients. While the chickpeas are slightly acid forming, the lemon juice, garlic, olive oil, and optional tahini help to balance them.

1	clove garlic
1	can (14 ounces) chickpeas (free of sodium, EDTA, sodium benzoate, or other chemicals), rinsed and drained
⅓	cup fresh lemon juice
2	tablespoons extra virgin olive oil
½	teaspoon unrefined sea salt
2	tablespoons tahini (optional)*

In a food processor, pulse the clove of garlic until it is minced. Add the chickpeas, lemon juice, oil, salt, and tahini, if using. Blend until creamy. Enjoy with vegetable crudités, as a sandwich spread, or atop a salad.

MAKES 6 SERVINGS

*Tahini is sesame puree. Choose a brand from your local health food store. It helps to alkalize this recipe and adds calcium, as tahini is rich in usable calcium.

VARIATIONS:

Roasted Red Pepper Hummus: Add 1 roasted and seeded red bell pepper with the garlic and pulse until finely chopped. Blend with the other ingredients.

Basil Hummus: Add a handful of fresh basil and pulse until the basil is mixed but not mashed into the hummus.

Warm Hummus: Warm and serve as a mashed potato–type side dish.

Spicy Chile Hummus: Add 1 chile pepper to the garlic (wear plastic gloves when handling) and pulse until minced. Add the remaining ingredients and blend together.

Per serving: 110 calories, 4 g protein, 13 g carbohydrates, 5 g total fat, 0.5 g saturated fat, 3 g fiber, 212 mg sodium

Roasted Red Pepper and Caramelized Onion Dip/Spread

Roasted red pepper and caramelized onion are two of my favorite ingredients. Combined, they are a flavor sensation. This dip/spread can be used with flatbreads, with crudités, on sandwiches, or in wraps.

1	tablespoon extra virgin olive oil
1	large red bell pepper
1	large onion, coarsely chopped
1	can (14 ounces) chickpeas, drained
1	cup fresh basil
½	teaspoon unrefined sea salt
	Pinch of ground red pepper
1	tablespoon water

In a medium skillet over low to medium heat, heat the oil. Add the whole red bell pepper, flipping it to cook all sides. Remove from the heat when cooked. Allow it to cool, then remove the seeds and stem.

Add the onion to the skillet and cook until lightly browned.

In a food processor, place the chickpeas, cooked red bell pepper, and cooked onion. Blend until coarsely chopped. Add the basil, salt, ground red pepper, and water and pulse until the basil is coarsely chopped and blended into the chickpea mixture.

MAKES 8 SERVINGS

Per serving: 63 calories, 2 g protein, 9 g carbohydrates, 2 g total fat, 0.5 g saturated fat, 2 g fiber, 157 mg sodium

Chunky Guacamole

This guacamole is a meal in itself. It is full of vegetables that add nutrition, alkalizing capacity, and tons of flavor. Enjoy it on top of mixed greens, with vegetable crudités, or on its own as a delicious avocado salad.

2	avocados, halved and pitted
1	tomato, finely chopped
1	red or yellow bell pepper, finely chopped
1	tablespoon finely chopped red onion
1	cup loosely packed fresh cilantro, finely chopped
½	jalapeño chile pepper (optional—wear plastic gloves when handling), finely chopped
1	lime, halved
½	teaspoon unrefined sea salt

Scoop the flesh from the avocados into a medium bowl and mash it. Add the tomato and bell pepper. Add the onion, cilantro, and chile pepper, if using, to the mixture. Squeeze fresh lime juice over the avocado mixture. Add the salt and stir together until well mixed.

MAKES 4 SERVINGS

Per serving: 182 calories, 3 g protein, 14 g carbohydrates, 15 g total fat, 2 g saturated fat, 8 g fiber, 307 mg sodium

Super Fat-Burning Salsa

Once you've tasted this delicious fresh salsa, you'll never go back to bottled versions. Not only does it taste great, but it also takes only about 5 minutes to make and is packed with nutrients that boost metabolism and burn fat. The garlic and onion improve the liver's ability to break down fats and detoxify harmful chemicals, the capsaicin in the jalapeño chile pepper fires up your metabolism, and the lime juice and tomatoes help balance your body chemistry in favor of alkalinity. But you'll quickly forget how healthy this salsa is once you taste it. It's one of my favorite foods. Serve it with celery sticks, over cooked quinoa or brown rice, or on organic corn tortilla shells.

1	clove garlic
½	small onion
½	jalapeño chile pepper (wear plastic gloves when handling)
2	large, ripe organic tomatoes, quartered
2	teaspoons fresh lime juice
1	teaspoon psyllium powder (a natural fiber that acts as a thickener)
	Pinch of Celtic sea salt or Himalayan crystal salt

In a food processor (I use a small one but any size will do), process the garlic, onion, and pepper until finely chopped. Add the tomatoes and pulse until they are coarsely chopped. Pour into a serving bowl, add the lime juice and psyllium powder, and mix together until all ingredients are combined. Allow the salsa to thicken for 10 minutes before serving. You can store it, covered, in the refrigerator for up to 3 days.

MAKES 2 SERVINGS

Per serving: 48 calories, 2 g protein, 11 g carbohydrates, 1 g total fat, 0 g saturated fat, 3 g fiber, 158 mg sodium

Soups

Angela's Hearty Minestrone Soup

This hearty soup from Angela Grow is perfect for a cold winter night but so good you'll want to enjoy it more often than that! It is delicious served with Basic Spelt Muffins (page 239). I followed Angela's recommendation to make an extra-large batch of minestrone since it is even better the next day. Also, it freezes well and can be stored for those days you just don't have the time or energy to make dinner.

1	onion, chopped
1	tablespoon coconut oil or palm oil
2–3	cloves garlic, finely chopped
1	can (28 ounces) diced tomatoes
1	small zucchini, chopped
1	cup chopped fresh green beans
1	teaspoon dried basil
1	teaspoon dried oregano
1	cup brown rice, spelt, or other whole grain pasta
1	can (15 ounces) kidney beans
1	can (15 ounces) chickpeas
6–8	cups water (depending on how "brothy" you like your soup)
	Sea salt and ground black pepper

In a large soup pot over medium heat, caramelize the onion in the oil, not allowing the oil to smoke. Briefly cook the garlic in the oil, stirring frequently. Add the tomatoes, zucchini, green beans, basil, oregano, rice or spelt or pasta, kidney beans, chickpeas, water, salt, and pepper. Let simmer until the rice, spelt, or pasta is tender, following package directions. Adjust the spices to taste.

MAKES 4 SERVINGS

Per serving: 380 calories, 16 g protein, 66 g carbohydrates, 5 g total fat, 3 g saturated fat, 12 g fiber, 765 mg sodium

Harvest Soup

My friend Dr. Cobi Slater shared this delicious recipe she developed.
Packed with veggies, and even a fruit (green apples), this unique soup is
the perfect blend of flavors. Be sure to choose a monosodium glutamate
(MSG)–free rotisserie chicken if you buy one from your local grocery
store. You'll love this soup.

8	cups chicken or vegetable broth
1	rotisserie chicken, deboned and cut into bite-size pieces
2	tablespoons extra virgin olive oil
1	onion, chopped
2	carrots, chopped
4	ribs celery, chopped
2	sweet potatoes, peeled and chopped
2	green apples, peeled and chopped
1	teaspoon unrefined sea salt
	Pinch of ground black pepper
½	cup apple cider
1	teaspoon dried basil
1	teaspoon parsley

In a large pot over medium heat, heat the chicken or vegetable broth until close
to boiling. Add the chicken and reduce the heat to a simmer.

In a medium pan over medium heat, heat the oil. Cook the onion, carrots, celery, and
sweet potatoes until soft. Add the apples and continue to cook, stirring frequently.
When the vegetables and apples are just cooked, add them to the broth.

Add the salt, pepper, cider, basil, and parsley and bring the soup to a boil. Reduce
the heat and let simmer for 20 minutes.

MAKES 4 SERVINGS

Per serving: 502 calories, 49 g protein, 40 g carbohydrates, 17 g total fat, 4 g saturated fat,
6 g fiber, 2,166 mg sodium

Hearty Beet-Quinoa Soup

This delicious soup, full of fiber and nutrients, is one of the simplest dishes to make. I throw everything but the quinoa into a slow cooker at night and add the quinoa 30 minutes before I'm ready to eat. Et voilà! *It's done. The quinoa adds protein, some good carbs, and fiber, making this a hearty meal in a bowl.*

4	carrots, chopped
1	large onion, chopped
3	ribs celery, peeled and chopped
3	beets, chopped
3	sprigs fresh thyme
2	sprigs fresh rosemary
8	cups water
1	teaspoon unrefined salt
1	(3") piece kelp (optional, but adds flavor and minerals to the soup)
½	cup quinoa

In a medium to large slow cooker, place the carrots, onion, celery, and beets. Add the thyme and rosemary. Pour in the water. Add the salt and kelp. Cover and cook on low for 6 to 8 hours or overnight. Half an hour to an hour before serving, add the quinoa to the hot soup, cover, and continue to cook on low.

MAKES 4 SERVINGS

Per serving: 151 calories, 5 g protein, 30 g carbohydrates, 2 g total fat, 0.5 g saturated fat, 6 g fiber, 726 mg sodium

Quick and Simple Black Bean Soup

One of Angela Grow's favorite recipes, this quick and simple black bean soup really lives up to its name. What the name doesn't tell you is how great it tastes. While it takes about 40 minutes for the rice to cook, the assembly time is only about 5 minutes, making it perfect when you just don't have much time to cook. How could anything so fast and easy taste so fantastic? You'll have to discover it for yourself. And unlike most soups, which lack much nutritional value, this one is packed with fiber and vegetables.

1	tablespoon coconut oil
1	onion, chopped
2	Anaheim chile peppers, chopped (wear plastic gloves when handling)
2–3	cloves garlic, minced
	Sea salt to taste
2	cans (15 ounces each) black beans, rinsed and drained
½	cup brown rice
2	cans (16 ounces each) diced tomatoes
6–8	cups water
1	teaspoon ground cumin
1	teaspoon chili powder (or use an MSG-free taco seasoning like Trader Joe's in place of the cumin and chili powder, if you prefer)
1	avocado, sliced, for garnish

In a large soup pot over medium heat, heat the oil. Cook the onion and peppers in the oil, stirring frequently, until they are caramelized. Add the garlic, salt, beans, rice, tomatoes, water, cumin, and chili powder. Bring to a boil and then simmer over medium heat until the rice is tender, about 40 minutes. Adjust the spices to taste. Serve garnished with the avocado.

MAKES 4 SERVINGS

Per serving: 293 calories, 11 g protein, 51 g carbohydrates, 5 g total fat, 3 g saturated fat, 9 g fiber, 968 mg sodium

Shrimp-Tomato Soup

Most soups, even those served in restaurants, are flavored with soup base that contains harmful MSG. This one gets its flavor from the shrimp, clam juice, and herbs. And it's packed full of flavor. It was created and shared by my Facebook friend Denise Passerello, a nutritionist and creator of the excellent Web site www.Fresh-Fitness.com. While it is acid forming, it offers many important nutrients such as the phytonutrient lycopene in the tomatoes, and the clam juice adds essential minerals to your diet.

3	tablespoons organic extra virgin coconut oil
1	large onion, finely chopped
4–5	cloves garlic, minced
1	cup chardonnay
1	bottle (8 ounces) clam juice
4	tomatoes, peeled and chopped
1	teaspoon sea salt
¾	teaspoon dried oregano
½	teaspoon freshly ground black pepper
1	pound small to medium shrimp, peeled and deveined
¼	cup chopped parsley

In a large pot over medium heat, heat the oil. Cook the onion and garlic, stirring frequently, for 5 minutes.

Add the chardonnay, clam juice, tomatoes, salt, oregano, and pepper. Bring to a boil, reduce the heat, and simmer for 20 minutes.

Stir in the shrimp and cook for 4 minutes. Stir in the parsley and serve.

MAKES 2 SERVINGS

Per serving: 607 calories, 50 g protein, 25 g carbohydrates, 26 g total fat, 19.5 g saturated fat, 5 g fiber, 1,780 mg sodium

Thai Ginger-Coconut Soup

This is one of my favorite soups. It is perfect for a cool autumn or winter dinner but so good you'll probably want to make it year-round. Your body will love the fat-fighting medium-chain triglycerides found in coconut milk and coconut oil. The lean chicken is an excellent source of protein, albeit an acid-forming one. The brown rice and vegetables provide good carbs and plenty of nutrients.

1	tablespoon coconut oil
1	cup brown rice
2	large carrots, chopped
2	ribs celery, chopped
1	large onion, chopped
3	cups water
½	fresh Thai chile pepper, chopped (wear plastic gloves when handling), or ¼ teaspoon dried
1	(2") piece fresh ginger, cut into matchsticks
1	5-ounce organic boneless, skinless chicken breast, thinly sliced
1	can (14 ounces) full-fat coconut milk
	Celtic sea salt or Himalayan crystal salt

In a large pot or Dutch oven over medium heat, melt the oil. Add the rice, carrots, celery, onion, water, pepper, and ginger to the pot. Cover and cook over medium heat for 30 minutes. If the soup starts to boil, reduce the heat. Add the chicken to the soup. Add the coconut milk and cook for another 15 minutes. Add salt to taste, and serve immediately.

MAKES 4 SERVINGS

Per serving: 467 calories, 14 g protein, 46 g carbohydrates, 27 g total fat, 22 g saturated fat, 5 g fiber, 180 mg sodium

Salads and Salad Dressings

60 Seconds to Slim Signature Salad

Topped with chicken, wild salmon, or chickpeas, this delicious salad has the perfect ratio of alkaline to acid ingredients. Enjoy it often!

1	boneless, skinless chicken breast or 1 (12-ounce) piece wild salmon (for a vegetarian alternative, substitute ½ cup cooked chickpeas)
1	carrot, grated
½	cucumber, grated
1	beet, grated
2	cups bean sprouts, washed
1	cup loosely packed fresh mint leaves, coarsely chopped
	Juice of ½ grapefruit
	Pinch of unrefined sea salt
2	tablespoons extra virgin olive oil
1	avocado, halved and sliced

In a covered skillet over medium heat, pan-fry the chicken or salmon, adding water as necessary. Cook 10 minutes on each side for the chicken and 5 minutes on each side for the salmon.

Meanwhile, in a large bowl, place the carrot, cucumber, and beet. Add the bean sprouts and the mint. In a jar with a lid, place the grapefruit juice, salt, and oil. Secure the lid and shake vigorously. Pour the dressing over the vegetables and toss. Divide the vegetable mixture between 2 plates. Cut the chicken or salmon in half and place 1 piece atop each plate. (Alternatively, add the chilled or gently warmed chickpeas to the vegetable mixture.) Top each plate with half of the avocado.

MAKES 2 SERVINGS

Per serving: 610 calories, 45 g protein, 33 g carbohydrates, 38 g total fat, 6 g saturated fat, 14 g fiber, 322 mg sodium

Alkalizing Cucumber Salad

Cucumbers are one of the most alkalizing vegetables. This simple salad is surprisingly delicious for the minimal amount of effort it requires. It takes about 5 to 10 minutes to throw together and is very alkalizing, making it a good choice when you need to push your pH in the right direction.

1	cucumber, sliced into 3″ spears
2	tablespoons fresh lime juice
¼	teaspoon unrefined sea salt

In a small to medium bowl, combine the cucumber, lime juice, and salt. Marinate for 5 to 10 minutes at room temperature to allow the flavors to mingle.

Serve as a side salad or atop mixed greens.

MAKES 2 SERVINGS

Per serving: 19 calories, 2 g protein, 4 g carbohydrates, 0 g total fat, 0 g saturated fat, 2 g fiber, 295 mg sodium

Balsamic Salmon Spinach Salad

Enliven your salads with this flavorful recipe created by Dr. Cobi Slater. Packed with anti-inflammatory essential fats, this salad is an excellent choice to take down the inflammation in your body, which can contribute to weight gain and illness. Both the wild salmon and the raw walnuts add protein and omega-3 fatty acids. Unlike farmed salmon, wild-caught salmon tends to be low in harmful toxins like mercury, making it a better choice. Even if you don't normally like the taste of walnuts, try raw, unsalted ones from your local health food store. I've had client after client come back and tell me that they never thought they'd like walnuts.

1	(12-ounce) wild salmon fillet
4	tablespoons balsamic vinaigrette
6	cups spinach
½	cup pitted and cubed avocado
2	tablespoons chopped raw, unsalted walnuts
2	tablespoons sunflower seeds
2	tablespoons unsulphured dried cranberries
1	cup halved cherry tomatoes

Preheat the broiler. On a baking sheet, place the salmon. Brush it with 2 tablespoons of the vinaigrette. Broil the salmon for 10 to 15 minutes, or until it flakes easily. Divide the salmon into 4 pieces.

In a large bowl, toss the spinach with the remaining 2 tablespoons of vinaigrette. Divide the spinach among 4 plates and top it with the avocado, walnuts, sunflower seeds, cranberries, tomatoes, and salmon.

MAKES 4 SERVINGS

Per serving: 257 calories, 20 g protein, 10 g carbohydrates, 16 g total fat, 2 g saturated fat, 3 g fiber, 172 mg sodium

Chicken and Peach Salad

The contrasting flavors of savory chicken and sweet peaches create a taste sensation. I'm so glad Dr. Cobi Slater shared this excellent recipe with me. The dressing is light and fresh tasting. While the vinegar, peaches, and chicken are acid forming, the mint, cucumber, and salad greens are alkalizing, which helps to offset the acidic ingredients.

3	peaches, peeled and cubed
2	cups cubed cooked chicken breast
1	cucumber, seeded and chopped
3	tablespoons finely chopped red onion
¼	cup white wine vinegar
1	tablespoon lemon juice
1	tablespoon agave nectar
⅓	cup chopped fresh mint
	Unrefined sea salt and ground black pepper
1	small container (10 ounces) mixed greens

In a large bowl, combine the peaches, chicken, cucumber, and onion. Set aside.

In a food processor or blender, combine the vinegar, lemon juice, agave nectar, mint, and salt and pepper. Process until smooth.

Drizzle the dressing over the chicken mixture.

Divide the salad greens evenly among 4 plates and spoon the chicken mixture over them.

MAKES 4 SERVINGS

Per serving: 217 calories, 24 g protein, 25 g carbohydrates, 3 g total fat, 1 g saturated fat, 3 g fiber, 128 mg sodium

Five-Spice Chicken and Orange Salad

The sweet, rich flavors of Chinese five-spice powder combine with the oranges and chicken for a taste explosion. I'm not even a big fan of oranges, and I love this salad. Developed by Dr. Cobi Slater, it's an excellent choice any time. Who said salad had to be boring? You'll never think that again after tasting this delicious dish. I could eat it every day.

SALAD

2	teaspoons extra virgin olive oil, divided
1	teaspoon Chinese five-spice powder (available in most health food stores)
½	teaspoon unrefined sea salt
½	teaspoon freshly ground black pepper
1	pound boneless, skinless chicken breasts
2	oranges
3	cups mixed wild greens
1	red bell pepper, chopped
½	cup thinly sliced red onion

DRESSING

1	orange
3	tablespoons apple cider vinegar
1	tablespoon Dijon mustard
4	teaspoons extra virgin olive oil
½	teaspoon unrefined sea salt
	Freshly ground black pepper

To make the salad: Preheat the oven to 450°F.

In a small bowl, combine 1 teaspoon of the oil, the five-spice powder, the salt, and the black pepper. Rub the mixture onto both sides of the chicken breasts.

In a large ovenproof nonstick skillet over medium-high heat, heat the remaining 1 teaspoon of the oil. Add the chicken breasts and cook until browned on one side, 3 to 5 minutes. Turn them over and transfer the pan to the oven. Roast until the chicken is just cooked through, 6 to 8 minutes. Set the chicken aside.

Meanwhile, over a large bowl, peel and segment the 2 oranges, collecting the segments and any juice in the bowl. Add the greens, bell pepper, and onion to the bowl.

To make the dressing: In a small bowl, grate the zest of the orange and then juice the orange.

In a medium bowl, whisk together the vinegar, mustard, oil, salt, and black pepper to taste. Add the orange zest and juice.

Pour the dressing over the large bowl of greens and toss to combine. Slice the chicken and add it to the salad.

MAKES 2 SERVINGS

Per serving: 791 calories, 52 g protein, 39 g carbohydrates, 49 g total fat, 7.5 g saturated fat, 7 g fiber, 1,648 mg sodium

Greek Quinoa Salad

This is one of my favorite foods. The quinoa and vegetables are alkalizing, plus unlike most grains, quinoa is high in protein, making it an excellent food for losing fat and building muscle. This salad can be made ahead and refrigerated for a quick and easy meal when you're short on time.

1	cup quinoa
1	teaspoon dried basil
½	teaspoon dried oregano
2	tablespoons fresh lemon juice
½	onion, finely chopped
1	tablespoon extra virgin olive oil
½	teaspoon unrefined sea salt
1	red bell pepper, chopped
½	cucumber, chopped

In a medium pot, cook the quinoa along with the basil and oregano, according to package instructions. Allow to cool. In a bowl, combine the lemon juice, onion, and olive oil. Add the salt to the lemon-onion mixture and set aside for 5 to 10 minutes. When the quinoa has cooled, add the pepper, cucumber, and the lemon-onion mixture. Toss together. Eat immediately or refrigerate for later.

MAKES 2 SERVINGS

Per serving: 415 calories, 14 g protein, 64 g carbohydrates, 12 g total fat, 1.5 g saturated fat, 9 g fiber, 608 mg sodium

My Favorite Greek Salad

With a name like that, you probably don't need me to tell you how good this salad is. It's packed with alkaline vegetables, digestion-boosting mint, and health-building phytonutrients such as lycopene, which has been shown to help prevent cancer. But it tastes so good you may forget how healthy it really is!

SALAD

1	large cucumber, chopped
3	tomatoes, chopped
1	large red bell pepper, chopped
½	small red onion, finely sliced
1	cup loosely packed fresh mint, finely chopped

GREEK SALAD DRESSING

2	tablespoons fresh lemon juice
¼	cup extra virgin olive oil
1	teaspoon dried basil
1	teaspoon dried oregano
½	teaspoon ground black pepper
½	teaspoon unrefined sea salt
	Pinch of ground red pepper

To make the salad: In a large bowl, combine the cucumber, tomatoes, and bell pepper. Add the onion and mint.

To make the dressing: In a screw-top jar or small food processor or blender, combine the lemon juice, olive oil, basil, oregano, ground black pepper, salt, and ground red pepper. Cover and shake or blend. Pour over the salad and let sit for at least 30 minutes to allow the flavors to combine.

MAKES 2 SERVINGS

Per serving: 356 calories, 5 g protein, 25 g carbohydrates, 29 g total fat, 4 g saturated fat, 9 g fiber, 620 mg sodium

Roasted Sweet Potato Salad

The roasted (actually, lightly pan-fried) sweet potatoes really boost this basic green salad. It's easy to make and even better to eat, and the sweetness of the potatoes provides a great contrast with the savory Cilantro Dressing. Yum!

SALAD

1	tablespoon coconut oil
1	small sweet potato, sliced into thin disks
	Pinch of unrefined sea salt
2–3	cups mixed salad greens

CILANTRO DRESSING

½	cup olive oil
2	tablespoons fresh lemon juice
	Pinch of unrefined sea salt
1	small clove garlic
½	cup loosely packed fresh cilantro

To make the salad: In a large skillet over low to medium heat, warm half of the coconut oil. Add as many of the sweet potato disks as will fit in a single layer. Sprinkle with the salt.

Cook until golden, and flip. Cook for another 5 minutes or until the sweet potato disks are cooked through. If necessary, cook additional sweet potato disks in another batch, following the same instructions.

To make the dressing: In a screw-top jar or small food processor or blender, combine the olive oil, lemon juice, salt, garlic, and cilantro. Cover and shake or blend together.

In a large bowl, toss the greens with the dressing. Place the greens in serving dishes, top with the sweet potato disks, and serve.

MAKES 2 SERVINGS

Per serving: 611 calories, 2 g protein, 17 g carbohydrates, 63 g total fat, 14 g saturated fat, 3 g fiber, 347 mg sodium

Asian Ginger Vinaigrette

I eat a lot of salads, so it's important to me to have variety. This dressing helps to keep salads interesting. I love the pungent gingery flavor with the sweetness of the honey and rice vinegar and the sweet-savory miso. Miso is a fermented soy (or sometimes brown rice) paste packed with healing and digestion-promoting enzymes. It has a unique but yummy flavor. This dressing can be made ahead and stored in a glass jar in the refrigerator. Toss it with greens or grated vegetables of your choice.

⅔   cup extra virgin olive oil (preferably a fruity-tasting type)

⅓   cup rice wine vinegar

3   teaspoons miso

1   teaspoon raw, unrefined honey

1   tablespoon grated fresh ginger

In a screw-top jar or blender, combine the oil, vinegar, miso, honey, and ginger. Cover and shake or blend until smooth. Toss over greens, grated vegetables, kelp noodles, or cooked spaghetti squash.

MAKES 8 SERVINGS

Per serving: 167 calories, 1 g protein, 2 g carbohydrates, 19 g total fat, 3 g saturated fat, 0.5 g fiber, 68 mg sodium

Savory Garlic Dressing

This is my favorite salad dressing. It's delicious served over salad greens or tossed with cooked greens like kale or collards. Either way, it makes greens taste amazing. Enjoy.

½   cup olive oil

2   tablespoons lemon juice

1   clove garlic, minced

1   teaspoon Dijon mustard

⅓   cup white wine vinegar

1   teaspoon unrefined sea salt

     Pinch of freshly cracked black pepper

     Pinch of ground red pepper

In a screw-top jar or blender, combine the oil, lemon juice, garlic, mustard, vinegar, salt, black pepper, and red pepper. Cover and shake or blend until smooth and creamy. Serve over romaine lettuce or cooked greens.

MAKES 8 SERVINGS

Per serving: 122 calories, 1 g protein, 1 g carbohydrates, 14 g total fat, 2 g saturated fat, 1 g fiber, 310 mg sodium

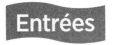

Black Bean Chili

Here is the recipe for my favorite chili. It is packed with nutritious veggies, black beans, and lean chicken or turkey, depending on your preference. This quick and delicious dinner can be made in 30 minutes (most of which is cooking time). It's so good your guests will never suspect it's healthy.

1	tablespoon olive oil
1	large carrot, chopped
1	large onion, chopped
2	ribs celery, chopped
1	pound organic 93% lean ground turkey or chicken
1	red bell pepper, coarsely chopped
1	jar (15 ounces) tomato sauce (preferably organic and free of sugar and additives)
½	teaspoon chili powder
2	teaspoons ground cumin
1	teaspoon dried basil
1	teaspoon unrefined sea salt
2	cans (15 ounces each) black beans, drained

In a large skillet over medium heat, warm the oil. Cook the carrot, onion, and celery, stirring frequently, until lightly browned. Add the turkey or chicken and cook, stirring frequently, until it is cooked through. Add the bell pepper, tomato sauce, chili powder, cumin, basil, and salt and mix thoroughly. Finally, add the beans to the mixture. Simmer for 20 minutes, or until all the vegetables are soft and the flavors have mingled.

MAKES 4 SERVINGS

Per serving: 381 calories, 31 g protein, 26 g carbohydrates, 15 g total fat, 3 g saturated fat, 11 g fiber, 1,340 mg sodium

Coconut Vegetable Curry

This curry, developed by Dr. Cobi Slater, is the perfect comfort food when you want a hearty meal that sticks to your ribs without sticking to your waistline. The spices not only add flavor but also help to balance bowel flora, which is important for weight loss and overall health.

2	tablespoons extra virgin olive oil
1	tablespoon chopped fresh ginger
1½	teaspoons cumin seeds
1	teaspoon black mustard seeds
3	small red potatoes, cubed
3	carrots, finely chopped
½	teaspoon ground turmeric
2	teaspoons ground coriander
1	teaspoon curry powder
1	tablespoon tomato paste
1	can (14 ounces) full-fat coconut milk
¼	cup water
2	small zucchini, finely chopped
1	cup frozen peas
2	cups chickpeas
1	teaspoon unrefined sea salt
½	cup chopped fresh cilantro
2	cups cooked brown rice or quinoa

In a large pot over medium heat, heat the oil. Cook the ginger, cumin seeds, and mustard seeds for 1 to 2 minutes, or until the seeds begin to pop.

Add the potatoes, carrots, turmeric, coriander, and curry powder. Stir well and continue to cook for another minute. Then add the tomato paste, coconut milk, and water. Stir well.

Simmer, covered, for 5 to 10 minutes, or until the potatoes and carrots are crisp-tender. Add the zucchini, peas, chickpeas, and salt. Cover the pot and simmer another 6 to 7 minutes, or until the vegetables are tender. Remove from the heat and stir in the cilantro.

Serve over brown rice or quinoa.

MAKES 4 SERVINGS

Per serving: 652 calories, 18 g protein, 82 g carbohydrates, 31 g total fat, 19.5 g saturated fat, 15 g fiber, 724 mg sodium

Ginger Broccoli and Tofu Stir-Fry

Okay, I know combining many people's most dreaded foods, broccoli and tofu, doesn't sound very appetizing, but somehow Dr. Cobi Slater developed a combination of flavors in this recipe that's dynamic. You'll never think of broccoli and tofu the same way again, which is probably a good thing. The Asian flavors in this dish are the perfect match for all these vegetables. Delish!

1	pound extra-firm tofu, drained
2	tablespoons tamari soy sauce
2	tablespoons extra virgin olive oil, divided
2	teaspoons minced scallions
2	teaspoons finely chopped fresh ginger
2	cloves garlic, minced
1	tablespoon arrowroot powder or cornstarch
¼	teaspoon red-pepper flakes
2	cups broccoli florets
2	cups sliced mushrooms
1	red bell pepper, cut into thin strips
¼	cup water
1	teaspoon sesame oil

Slice the tofu into cubes. In a bowl, toss them with the soy sauce. Set aside for 5 to 10 minutes.

In a wok or large nonstick skillet, heat 1 tablespoon of the olive oil over high heat. When the oil is hot, lower the heat to medium-high and stir-fry the scallions, ginger, and garlic for 30 seconds.

Drain the tofu, reserving the soy sauce. Stir-fry the tofu in the wok for 2 minutes. Remove and set aside.

In a small bowl, using a fork or small whisk, mix the reserved soy sauce with the arrowroot powder or cornstarch and red-pepper flakes. Set aside.

In the wok, over high heat, heat the remaining 1 tablespoon of the olive oil. Stir-fry the broccoli, mushrooms, and bell pepper for 2 minutes.

Add the water and bring to a boil. Cover the wok and reduce the heat to medium. Steam the vegetables for 5 minutes, or until slightly tender. Add the sesame oil, reserved soy sauce–arrowroot mixture, and reserved tofu. Cook until the sauce thickens. Serve immediately.

MAKES 2 SERVINGS

Per serving: 512 calories, 31 g protein, 22 g carbohydrates, 36 g total fat, 5 g saturated fat, 8 g fiber, 976 mg sodium

Grilled Chicken with Citrus Salsa

This citrus salsa adds a fresh, vibrant flavor to grilled chicken. It's another delicious, nutritious, and easy-to-make recipe from Dr. Cobi Slater. The grapefruit, orange, scallions, cherry tomatoes, lime, and cilantro create an explosion of flavor. This recipe is perfect for a hot summer night but is so good you'll want to make it year-round. I love it.

¼   cup lime juice, divided

3   tablespoons extra virgin olive oil, divided

4   boneless, skinless chicken breasts

     Pinch of unrefined sea salt

     Pinch of ground black pepper

1   orange, peeled and cut into small pieces

1   pink grapefruit, peeled and cut into small pieces

4   scallions, thinly sliced

10   cherry tomatoes, halved

     Zest and juice of ½ orange

     Zest of ½ lime

1   jalapeño chile pepper, finely chopped (wear plastic gloves when handling)

¼   cup chopped fresh cilantro

2   tomatillos, finely chopped

4   cups salad greens

Preheat the grill.

In a shallow dish, combine 3 tablespoons of the lime juice and 2 tablespoons of the oil. Rub the chicken with the salt and black pepper and add it to the marinade. Marinate for at least 20 minutes.

In a medium bowl, combine the orange, grapefruit, scallions, tomatoes, orange zest and juice, lime zest, chile pepper, cilantro, tomatillos, and the remaining 1 tablespoon of lime juice and 1 tablespoon of oil. Mix and set aside.

Remove the chicken from the marinade. Cook on the hot grill for 6 minutes on each side, or until a thermometer inserted in the thickest portion registers 165°F and the juices run clear. Remove the chicken from the grill and let stand a few minutes.

Divide the salad greens among 4 plates. Slice the chicken and arrange it on top of the greens. Spoon the salsa over each salad and serve.

MAKES 4 SERVINGS

Per serving: 304 calories, 28 g protein, 19 g carbohydrates, 14 g total fat, 2 g saturated fat, 4 g fiber, 230 mg sodium

Mediterranean Chicken

You'll love this Italian-inspired recipe from Dr. Cobi Slater. You can make the sauce in advance so it's a quick and easy meal when you're short on time. The flavors only get better as they mingle. It can be kept in the fridge for up to 2 weeks or in the freezer for up to 6 months. It's the perfect dish when you're craving Italian food, without all the carbs. Yum!

3	tablespoons extra virgin olive oil, divided
1	red onion, finely chopped
2	cups chopped plum tomatoes
¼	cup chicken or vegetable stock
2	cloves fresh garlic, minced
½	teaspoon dried basil
½	teaspoon dried oregano
¼	teaspoon dried thyme
¼	teaspoon finely crumbled bay leaf
¼	teaspoon coriander seeds
¼	teaspoon fennel seeds
4	boneless, skinless chicken breasts

In a large skillet over medium heat, heat 1 tablespoon of the oil.

Cook the onion, stirring frequently, until golden. Stir in the tomatoes, chicken or vegetable stock, garlic, basil, oregano, thyme, bay leaf, coriander seeds, and fennel seeds and simmer for 30 minutes. Remove from the heat.

In a separate large skillet over medium-high heat, heat the remaining 2 tablespoons of oil. Cook the chicken, uncovered, for 3 minutes per side or until a thermometer inserted in the thickest portion registers 165°F and the juices run clear.

Serve the chicken on 4 plates. Top with the sauce.

MAKES 4 SERVINGS

Per serving: 257 calories, 27 g protein, 7 g carbohydrates, 14 g total fat, 2 g saturated fat, 2 g fiber, 170 mg sodium

Fantastic Fish Tacos

This is the perfect way to add fish to your diet even if you're not much of a fish fan. The seasonings provide delicious flavor. The cabbage, sprouts, and salsa add texture, taste, and superb nutrition. They include plentiful amounts of enzymes to reduce the burden on your own stores. Developed by Dr. Cobi Slater, these tacos are perfect when you are tired of the same old food and want something exciting for dinner, but still want to maintain your waistline.

1½	pounds halibut, skinned and cut into 1" pieces
4	tablespoons fresh lime juice
3	cloves garlic, minced
1	jalapeño chile pepper, finely chopped (wear plastic gloves when handling)
2	teaspoons ground cumin
1	teaspoon seasoning salt (such as Herbamare)
2	tablespoons extra virgin olive oil
4	spelt or sprouted corn tortillas
2	cups thinly sliced napa cabbage
1	cup sprouts of your choice (such as mung bean sprouts, red clover sprouts, alfalfa sprouts)
1	cup Super Fat-Burning Salsa (page 255)

In a shallow dish, place the fish.

In a food processor, combine the lime juice, garlic, pepper, cumin, and seasoning salt. Blend for 1 minute.

Pour the marinade over the fish and marinate for at least 1 hour.

In a large skillet, heat the oil and cook the fish, stirring frequently, for 4 minutes. If needed, cook the fish in two batches.

Serve on the tortillas with the cabbage, sprouts, and salsa.

MAKES 4 SERVINGS

Per serving: 343 calories, 38 g protein, 20 g carbohydrates, 12 g total fat, 1.5 g saturated fat, 4 g fiber, 487 mg sodium

Open-Faced Veggie Sandwich

This is an easy and protein-packed lunch that takes only minutes to prepare, making it a go-to meal when you don't have much time or need something to grab and take with you.

2	tablespoons Hummus (page 252)
1	slice sprouted whole grain bread or gluten-free bread
1	avocado, sliced
1	red onion, sliced
1	tomato, sliced
1	cucumber, sliced
	Sea salt and ground black pepper
	Sunflower seeds

Spread the hummus on the slice of bread (sometimes I toast the bread first). Assemble the avocado, onion, tomato, and cucumber on top. Sprinkle with salt, pepper, and sunflower seeds, and enjoy! You may need a knife and fork to tackle this open-faced sandwich. Use your imagination when choosing veggies for this sandwich—if it is appealing to you, you are more likely to love eating it!

MAKES 1

Per sandwich: 551 calories, 15 g protein, 61 g carbohydrates, 32 g total fat, 4.5 g saturated fat, 24 g fiber, 470 mg sodium

Protein-Packed Burrito Bowl for One

This is a super-easy and refreshing meal, and you won't miss the cheese or sour cream. Angela Grow, the developer of this recipe, says her kids regularly ask for this for lunch. Another way to save time is to cook extra brown rice or quinoa and keep it in the refrigerator so that you can use it as you need to throughout the week.

1	cup cooked brown rice or quinoa
½	cup cooked pinto beans, black beans, or other beans of your choice
1	avocado, sliced
½	cup Super Fat-Burning Salsa (page 255)
1	cup finely chopped fresh greens
	Black olives, for garnish
	Chopped fresh cilantro, for garnish
	Dash of hot sauce
2	tablespoons fresh lemon juice

In a bowl, layer the rice or quinoa, beans, avocado, salsa, and greens (I prefer kale). Garnish with the black olives and cilantro, and add the hot sauce and lemon juice.

MAKES 1

Per bowl: 719 calories, 20 g protein, 97 g carbohydrates, 33 g total fat, 5 g saturated fat, 28 g fiber, 498 mg sodium

Vegan Enchilada Casserole

This is another delicious and wholesome meal from Angela Grow that's quick to make and full of fiber and vegetables. I love that it is a one-dish meal that saves preparation and cleanup time. But your tastebuds will love the incredible flavors.

1	onion, chopped
2	Anaheim chile peppers, chopped (wear plastic gloves when handling)
1	tablespoon coconut oil or palm oil
½	teaspoon ground cumin
1	can (15 ounces) black beans or pinto beans, drained and rinsed
1	can (15 ounces) enchilada or tomato sauce (be sure it contains no artificial flavors)
12	organic or sprouted corn tortillas (use only organic corn since almost all other corn is genetically modified and not a healthy option)
1	can (15 ounces) black olives, drained and sliced
	Finely chopped avocado, for garnish
	Chopped tomato, for garnish
	Jalapeño chile peppers, for garnish (optional—wear plastic gloves when handling)
	Cilantro, for garnish

Preheat the oven to 350°F.

In a skillet over medium heat, caramelize the onion and Anaheim chile peppers in the oil. Add the cumin and beans.

In a 13" × 9" baking dish, begin layering the ingredients. First, put a small amount of enchilada sauce in the bottom of the dish. Next, lay out several of the tortillas, then spoon the bean mixture over the tortillas, and finish with more enchilada sauce. Repeat this process until you have made 3 layers. Spread the olives over the top.

Place, uncovered, in the oven for 30 minutes, or until warmed through and bubbly. Garnish with the avocado, tomato, jalapeño chile peppers (if using), and cilantro.

MAKES 4 SERVINGS

Per serving: 387 calories, 9 g protein, 59 g carbohydrates, 12 g total fat, 3 g saturated fat, 10 g fiber, 1,032 mg sodium

Baked Maple Acorn Squash

I love autumn. I love the apple picking and the pumpkin patches. I love the cooler nights. This is the perfect dish on one of those cool autumn evenings. The recipe calls for acorn squash, but you can use other types of squash as well. This dish is packed with healing carotenes like beta-carotene that form vitamin A in your body. It's delicious served on its own as a side dish, or it can be filled with Cranberry Quinoa (page 291) for a lovely presentation.

1	acorn squash, halved lengthwise and seeded
1	teaspoon olive oil
½	teaspoon maple syrup
½	teaspoon palm sugar or coconut sap
	Pinch of unrefined salt

Preheat the oven to 350°F. On a small baking sheet, set the squash halves cut-side up. Puncture the flesh in a few places with a fork. Brush the exposed surfaces of the squash with the oil. Drizzle with the maple syrup. Sprinkle the palm sugar or coconut sap and the salt over the squash. Bake for 1 hour, or until the squash is tender.

MAKES 2 SERVINGS

Per serving: 115 calories, 2 g protein, 25 g carbohydrates, 3 g total fat, 0.5 g saturated fat, 3 g fiber, 154 mg sodium

Garlicky Greens

One of the most common questions I am asked is, "How can I cook greens to make them taste good?" Every time I give people these instructions, they come back and tell me they can't believe how good these greens taste. You can make this recipe using spinach, kale, collard greens, beet greens, or any other type of greens. Kale is my favorite since it is packed with minerals and grows easily even in northern climates. In addition to lots of alkalizing calcium, it contains a fair amount of fiber. And you can tell from its green color that it is packed with chlorophyll too. Somehow the combination of garlic and lemon juice makes fresh greens taste fantastic.

1   tablespoon coconut oil or extra virgin olive oil

1   large bunch kale (or other leafy green, if you prefer), stems removed, washed, and coarsely chopped

1   clove garlic, minced

2   tablespoons fresh lemon juice

Pinch of Himalayan crystal salt or Celtic sea salt

In a large skillet with a lid, heat the oil, being careful not to allow it to smoke. Add the kale to the skillet with a small amount of water. Cover and cook 3 minutes, or until the kale has turned a bright shade of green and softened. Add the garlic and cook, stirring frequently, for an additional minute or two. Remove from the heat and toss the kale with the lemon juice and salt. Serve immediately.

MAKES 2 SERVINGS

Per serving: 132 calories, 5 g protein, 15 g carbohydrates, 8 g total fat, 6 g saturated fat, 3 g fiber, 206 mg sodium

Crunchy Veggie Stir-Fry

Angela Grow shared this delicious stir-fry recipe with me. It is quick, easy, and packed full of nutrients. The idea is to not overcook the veggies—the crunchier, the better. The sky is the limit as far as what veggies you can use, so go ahead and throw in whatever you love and have available!

1	red bell pepper, sliced
1	yellow bell pepper, sliced
1	cup sliced mushrooms
1	medium onion, sliced
½	head of cabbage, thinly sliced
1	cup chopped broccoli
1	cup chopped asparagus
½	cup sliced carrots
3	cloves garlic, minced
2	tablespoons tamari soy sauce
1–3	tablespoons sesame oil
	Sliced raw almonds, for garnish (optional)

In a large skillet over medium heat, toss the bell peppers, mushrooms, onion, cabbage, broccoli, asparagus, carrots, and garlic until slightly cooked and warmed throughout. (There is no need for oil, but you can use a little grape seed oil or coconut oil, if desired.)

In a small bowl, combine the soy sauce and sesame oil to make a stir-fry sauce. Pour the sauce over the veggies and cook 1 minute longer. Garnish with the almonds, if desired. You can serve this over cooked brown rice or quinoa for a main-dish meal.

MAKES 2 SERVINGS

Per serving: 236 calories, 11 g protein, 37 g carbohydrates, 8 g total fat, 1 g saturated fat, 12 g fiber, 1,020 mg sodium

Edamame Stir-Fry

If you've never tried edamame (fresh, green soybeans), this recipe from
Dr. Cobi Slater is a great place to start. It can be whipped up in 10 minutes.
The flavors are excellent. It's the dish to make when you are bored with the
"same-old, same-old" foods.

1	cup frozen, shelled edamame
¼	cup coconut milk, divided
2	cloves garlic, minced
1	tablespoon grated fresh ginger
1	tablespoon red curry paste
2	cups chopped broccoli
1	yellow bell pepper, finely chopped
½	cup vegetable broth
¼	cup water
1	tablespoon tamari soy sauce
½	cup cherry tomatoes
2	scallions, chopped
1	tablespoon lime juice

In a medium saucepan, in enough water to cover, boil the edamame for 4 minutes. Drain and set aside.

In a large wok over high heat, heat 2 tablespoons of the coconut milk for 30 seconds, or until it boils. Stir in the garlic, ginger, and curry paste. Add the broccoli and pepper and stir-fry for 1 minute. Add the broth and water and stir-fry 2 minutes more. Stir in the soy sauce and the remaining coconut milk. Add the tomatoes, scallions, and reserved edamame and stir-fry until heated through. Drizzle with the lime juice. Serve immediately.

MAKES 2 SERVINGS

Per serving: 237 calories, 16 g protein, 24 g carbohydrates, 10 g total fat, 5.5 g saturated fat, 8 g fiber, 934 mg sodium

Basic Quinoa

Quinoa is delicious on its own, as a breakfast cereal with coconut or almond milk and flaxseeds, seasoned with fresh herbs, topped with vegetables, or as a warm or cold salad. It's quick, versatile, nutritious, delicious, high in protein, gluten free, and alkalizing! If you haven't been eating quinoa, you might want to start now. Here's the basic recipe for cooking quinoa.

1	cup quinoa
1½	cups water or broth

In a small pot, combine the quinoa and water or broth. Bring to a boil. Cover. Reduce the heat and cook for 15 to 20 minutes, or until the water is absorbed.

MAKES 4 SERVINGS

Per serving: 156 calories, 6 g protein, 27 g carbohydrates, 3 g total fat, 0.5 g saturated fat, 3 g fiber, 6 mg sodium

Cranberry Quinoa

Tired of the same old grain dishes? I was too—that's why I created cranberry quinoa. The cranberries add a great contrasting taste to the savory ingredients. It is delicious on its own or served in either Baked Maple Acorn Squash (page 286) or baked red or green bell peppers for a beautiful presentation.

1	cup quinoa
1½	cups water
2	tablespoons coconut oil
1	large onion, chopped
1	cup frozen or fresh cranberries
½	teaspoon dried basil
	Pinch of ground red pepper
1	teaspoon palm sugar or coconut sap
1	clove garlic, minced

In a small saucepan, combine the quinoa and water. Bring to a boil, then cover, reduce the heat to low, and cook for 15 to 20 minutes, or until the water is absorbed.

In the meantime, in a skillet over low to medium heat, cook the oil and onion until the onion is slightly brown, being careful not to let the oil smoke. Add the cranberries, basil, pepper, and palm sugar or coconut sap. Cook, stirring frequently, until the cranberries are heated through. Add the garlic to the onion-cranberry mixture and cook, stirring frequently, for a few minutes. Add the cooked quinoa and toss until all the ingredients are thoroughly mixed.

MAKES 4 SERVINGS

Per serving: 247 calories, 7 g protein, 35 g carbohydrates, 10 g total fat, 6 g saturated fat, 5 g fiber, 8 mg sodium

Farmers' Market Quinoa

This recipe is a great way to use vegetables you have in your fridge. Don't be afraid to use whichever ones you have on hand, as the recipe is quite versatile. This dish can be served warm, at room temperature, or cold over a plate of salad greens. Either way, it is delicious, fresh, and colorful. It can also be served with fresh bean sprouts and garnished with a sprig of cilantro.

1	tablespoon coconut oil
1	stem broccoli, peeled and finely chopped
1	large carrot, finely chopped
1	rib celery, finely chopped
½	onion, finely chopped
1	cup quinoa
½	teaspoon unrefined sea salt
2	cups water
½	red bell pepper, finely chopped
½	yellow or orange bell pepper, finely chopped
1	cup loosely packed cilantro leaves, coarsely chopped + 1 sprig for garnish
2	tablespoons fresh lime juice
	Handful of bean sprouts (optional)

In a medium pot over low to medium heat, place the coconut oil. Add the broccoli, carrot, celery, and onion. Cook for 5 minutes to slightly soften the vegetables, being careful not to allow the oil to smoke. Add the quinoa, salt, and water. Bring to a boil, then reduce the heat and simmer, covered, over low heat for 20 minutes, or until the water is absorbed into the quinoa.

In the meantime, in a medium serving bowl, place the peppers, cilantro, and lime juice. When the quinoa is finished, allow it to cool. Then mix the quinoa into the pepper-cilantro mixture. Toss to coat. Top with the bean sprouts, if using, and garnish with the sprig of cilantro before serving.

MAKES 4 SERVINGS

Per serving: 223 calories, 8 g protein, 36 g carbohydrates, 7 g total fat, 3 g saturated fat, 6 g fiber, 334 mg sodium

Pineapple-Basil Quinoa

Pineapple is loaded with natural sugars, so it's not a great weight-loss food. But this recipe has only a small amount of pineapple to add flavor without a lot of sugar. Along with the basil, it gives this quinoa dish an incredible taste.

1	cup quinoa
1½	cups water
2	tablespoons coconut oil, divided
1	cup fresh basil leaves
¾	cup finely chopped fresh pineapple
½	teaspoon Himalayan crystal salt or Celtic sea salt

In a small to medium pot, combine the quinoa, water, and 1 tablespoon of the oil. Bring to a boil. Once the water begins to boil, immediately reduce the heat to low and let simmer, covered, for 15 to 20 minutes, or until all the water has been absorbed.

In a medium to large bowl, toss together the cooked quinoa, the remaining 1 tablespoon of oil, the basil, pineapple, and salt until combined. Serve immediately.

MAKES 4 SERVINGS

Per serving: 231 calories, 6 g protein, 31 g carbohydrates, 9 g total fat, 6 g saturated fat, 3 g fiber, 104 mg sodium

Desserts

Strawberry Coconut Milk Ice Cream

My friend Angela Grow created this recipe for her husband, Bobby, a cancer survivor. She wanted a treat he could indulge in on occasion that wasn't too high in sugar, since she knew sugar compromises the immune system and increases acidity. This delightful ice cream is the result of her innovation. While it is still acid forming, it is an excellent treat to enjoy once in a while. The strawberries contain vitamin C and lots of healing phytonutrients, while the coconut milk provides healthy medium-chain triglycerides that help reset the thyroid gland and speed metabolism. As with all treats, enjoy in moderation and only on occasion.

2	cups fresh or frozen strawberries
1	can (14 ounces) full-fat coconut milk
2	tablespoons organic maple syrup
¼	teaspoon vanilla-flavored liquid stevia

In a blender, combine the strawberries, coconut milk, maple syrup, and stevia. Blend until thoroughly combined. Transfer to an ice cream maker for 20 to 25 minutes. (Follow the manufacturer's directions.) Serve immediately.

MAKES 4 SERVINGS

Per serving: 235 calories, 2 g protein, 14 g carbohydrates, 21 g total fat, 18.5 g saturated fat, 2 g fiber, 14 mg sodium

Angela's Spelt Pumpkin Scones

If you like scones, you'll love these vegan ones created by Angela Grow. The palm sugar or coconut sap adds sweetness without too many grams of sugar, making for mouthwatering scones.

2	cups spelt flour (you may substitute a gluten-free flour, if you prefer, but double the amount of flaxseeds and water)
¼	cup palm sugar or coconut sap
1	tablespoon aluminum-free baking powder
½	teaspoon sea salt
1	teaspoon ground cinnamon
½	teaspoon ground nutmeg
¼	teaspoon ground cloves
¼	teaspoon ground ginger
½	cup chopped raw, unsalted walnuts or pecans (optional)
6	tablespoons coconut oil, chilled
½	cup canned pumpkin
3	tablespoons almond milk
½	teaspoon vanilla-flavored liquid stevia
1	tablespoon ground flaxseeds mixed with 3 tablespoons water (allow to sit until it forms a gel)

Preheat the oven to 425°F.

In a large bowl, combine the flour, palm sugar or coconut sap, baking powder, salt, cinnamon, nutmeg, cloves, ginger, and walnuts or pecans, if using. Using a fork or pastry blender, combine the oil and dry ingredients until they resemble a coarse mixture.

In a separate bowl, combine the pumpkin, almond milk, stevia, and flaxseed mixture.

Next, add the pumpkin mixture to the flour mixture. Mix until a soft dough forms. Turn the dough onto a lightly floured surface and pat it into a 1"-thick circle that is 6" in diameter. Using a knife, cut the dough into 8 equal parts. On a lightly greased baking sheet, place the scones. Bake for 12 to 15 minutes. Remove from the oven and cool on a wire rack.

MAKES 8

Per scone: 245 calories, 5 g protein, 30 g carbohydrates, 12 g total fat, 9 g saturated fat, 5 g fiber, 318 mg sodium

Strawberry-Rhubarb Crisp

I love rhubarb but can rarely come up with enough recipes to use it all when I buy it or grow it in my garden. It's naturally high in fiber and low in sugar, so you can enjoy it in moderation while losing weight. Try pouring almond milk over leftovers from this recipe for an occasional breakfast treat.

3	cups chopped fresh rhubarb
3	cups sliced fresh strawberries
1	cup palm sugar or coconut sap, divided
1	cup sorghum flour, spelt flour, or brown rice flour
1	cup gluten-free oats
1	teaspoon ground cinnamon
½	teaspoon ground nutmeg
½	cup coconut oil

Preheat the oven to 350°F. Coat a 13" × 9" baking pan with cooking spray.

In a large bowl, toss the rhubarb and strawberries with ½ cup of the palm sugar or coconut sap. Pour the mixture into the baking pan. In a separate bowl, combine the flour, oats, cinnamon, nutmeg, and the remaining ½ cup of palm sugar or coconut sap. Use a fork to mix the oil into the flour mixture. Pour the flour mixture over the fruit mixture. Bake for 30 to 45 minutes, or until the fruit is bubbly.

MAKES 4 SERVINGS

Variation: You can substitute apples or berries for the rhubarb and strawberries in this dessert, depending on what's in season.

Per serving: 678 calories, 9 g protein, 98 g carbohydrates, 30 g total fat, 24 g saturated fat, 9 g fiber, 6 mg sodium

Banana Fudgesicles

This is the perfect dessert on a hot day when you don't want to bake but also want a sweet treat. They take only a few minutes to prepare but need several hours to freeze, so you'll want to make them in advance.

1   cup almond milk

1½   tablespoons unsweetened cocoa powder

1   frozen banana, sliced into ½"-thick pieces

1   teaspoon palm sugar or coconut sap

In a blender, combine the almond milk, cocoa, banana, and palm sugar or coconut sap. Blend until smooth, then pour into 4 ice pop molds. Add sticks at the appropriate time, following your mold manufacturer's directions. (Some manufacturers allow you to insert the sticks immediately, while others require some freezing first.)

MAKES 4

Per fudgesicle: 50 calories, 1 g protein, 11 g carbohydrates, 1 g total fat, 0 g saturated fat, 2 g fiber, 38 mg sodium

Conclusion

I had a client come to me a few years ago who declared that my program didn't work. I was surprised to hear this because I'd had many other people tell me how effective my program is, not just for weight loss but in reversing many serious health conditions, even supposedly incurable ones. I know from experience that it works.

I asked her what she was eating and was surprised to hear how many unhealthy foods she continued to include in her diet—foods that were not part of the food list I had provided. I asked her what she was drinking and discovered that, not only had she not cut back on her three cups of coffee daily, but that she was also still drinking alcoholic beverages, even though they are highly acid forming and feed pathogens in the bowels.

I asked her if she was taking the supplements I suggested, and she said, "Yes, of course." I asked her if she was taking anything else, and she proceeded to tell me about all the other supplements that so-called experts in her community had recommended, most of which were full of garbage ingredients, and the rest of which were either ineffective or actually thwarting her efforts to become more alkaline. I also learned that she was "too busy" even to walk regularly, or at all. After this assessment, I proceeded to tell her, "*Your* program doesn't work. I would encourage you to try *mine*."

I share this story because I'm sure there will be some readers who think this program doesn't work. If you find yourself not getting the results you'd like or actually having problems you're attributing to the program, please reread The Essential Plan and review Week 1 to see if there are ways you might be able to take your alkalizing efforts further. Of course, no one is perfect. But before you give up or conclude that you're not getting the results you want, I encourage you to check in with the program to see how closely yours matches mine. It's easy to fall back into bad habits, and it takes some effort and time to create new ones.

The 60 Seconds to Slim Plan is designed to help you lose excess weight. You can stay on the program after you've reached your target weight if you want to, or you can ease up on it a bit. That's up to your preference. Most people find that once they feel so much lighter, more vibrant, and energetic and experience fewer nagging health symptoms, they don't want to give up on the program. They may enjoy an occasional break from it for a night out or social situation and then get right back on it. But that's up to you.

I encourage you to follow this alkalizing program as best as you can to maintain the healthy weight you achieve and to enjoy better health. We only get one body in this life, so it's important to care for its needs. It will allow us greater freedom and energy to fully embrace life. Clarissa Pinkoa Estés said it so well in her book *Women Who Run with the Wolves:*

> The body is like an Earth. It is a land unto itself. It is as vulnerable to overbuilding, being carved into pieces, cut off, overmined, and short of its power as any landscape. We tend to think of the body as this "other" that does its thing without us. Many people treat their bodies as if the body were a slave. We have only to pay heed to our bodies to know what we must do. The body is not sculpture or marble. Its purpose is to protect, contain, support, and fire the spirit and soul within it, to be a repository for memory, to fill us with feeling. It is to lift us and propel us, to prove that we exist, that we are here, to give us grounding, heft, weight. The body is best understood as a being in its own right, one who loves us, depends on us, one to whom we are sometimes mother, and who sometimes is mother to us.

Keep your body moving, nourish it, rest it, rebuild it, and care for it and it will reciprocate with a lighter version of you, increased vitality, and improved health.

Wishing you great health,
Michelle Schoffro Cook, PhD, ROHP

About the Author

Michelle Schoffro Cook, PhD, RNCP, ROHP

Dr. Schoffro Cook is an international bestselling author whose 13 works include *The Ultimate pH Solution, The 4-Week Ultimate Body Detox Plan, The Phytozyme Cure,* and *Allergy-Proof.* Her books have been translated into many languages, including Spanish, Greek, Chinese, and Indonesian.

She holds a PhD in traditional natural medicine, a master's of science in natural health, a bachelor of science degree in holistic nutrition, and a diploma of orthomolecular nutrition. With over two decades of experience in the nutrition and natural health field, Dr. Schoffro Cook is a registered nutritional consulting practitioner, registered orthomolecular health practitioner, Reiki Master, Reconnective Healing Practitioner, and bioenergetic medicine practitioner.

Dr. Schoffro Cook received the World Leading Intellectual Award for her contribution to natural medicine, a Forty Under 40 Award, a Crystal Communicator Award, and numerous other communications awards. She has made over 1,000 media appearances, including being featured on or in *Woman's World, First for Women, YOU: The Owner's Manual Radio Show, Natural Solutions,* Oxygen, *Hello! Canada, Glow, Vegetarian Times,* and the Huffington Post. She is a regular blogger for Care2.com and WorldsHealthiestDiet.com.

Dr. Michelle Schoffro Cook is a member of the International Organization of Nutrition Consultants. Subscribe to her free e-magazine at www.WorldsHealthiestDiet.com. Learn more about her work at www.DrMichelleCook.com.

Endnotes

Introduction

1   Reuters, "75% of Americans Forecast to Be Overweight," *Vancouver Sun*, July 19, 2007, p. A9.

2   Joseph Mercola, DO, "What Started the Obesity Epidemic in America?" http://articles. mercola.com/sites/articles/archive/2011/07/26/what-caused-america-to-go-from-fit-to-fat.aspx, accessed July 26, 2011.

3   Ibid.

4   Ibid.

Chapter 1

1   Robert O. Young, "You Are Not Over-Weight—You Are Over-Acid."

2   Michelle Schoffro Cook, PhD, *The Ultimate pH Solution* (New York: Harper Collins, 2008).

3   David A. Bushinsky, MD, "Acid-Base Imbalance and the Skeleton," *European Journal of Nutrition* 40, no. 5 (October 2001): 238–244.

Chapter 2

1   "7 of the Most Unhealthy and Potentially Cancer-Causing Foods." http://renegadehealth. com/blog/2012/05/21/7-of-the-most-unhealthy-and-potentially-cancer-causing-foods, accessed September 6, 2012.

2   Colleen Doyle, MS, RD, "Hot Dog! Headlines Can Be Deceiving." http://www.cancer. org/Cancer/News/ExpertVoices/post/2011/03/31/Hot-dog!-HeadLines-Can-Be-Deceiving. aspx, accessed September 6, 2012.

3   Joseph Mercola, DO, "How Many Pounds Does One Extra Soft Drink Add to Your Body?" http://articles.mercola.com/sites/articles/archive/2006/08/24/how-many-pounds-does-one-extra-soft-drink-add-to-your-body.aspx, accessed September 6, 2012.

4   Lynne Melcombe, *Health Hazards of White Sugar* (Vancouver, BC: Alive Books, 2002).

5   "The Importance of Detoxification." Informational brochure. Advanced Nutrition Publications, Inc., 2002.

6   Patricia Fitzgerald, *The Detox Solution* (Santa Monica, CA: Illumination Press, 2001), p. 28.

7   Robert O. Young and Shelley Redford Young, *The pH Miracle for Weight Loss* (New York: Grand Central Life & Style, 2006).

8   Ibid.

9   Francine Larson, "We're Not Calves, Should We Be Drinking Cow's Milk?" http://www. examiner.com/article/we-re-not-calves-should-we-be-drinking-cow-s-milk-cancer-risk, accessed September 6, 2012.

10 Ibid.

Chapter 3

1   D. I. Jalal et al., "Increased fructose associates with elevated blood pressure," *Journal of the American Society of Nephrology,* September 2010. http://www.ncbi.nlm.nih.gov/pubmed/20595676, accessed April 30, 2012.

2   M. B. Abou-Donia, "Splenda alters gut microflora and increases intestinal p-glycoprotein and cytochrome p-450 in male rats," *Journal of Toxicology and Environmental Health,* 2008. http://www.ncbi.nlm.nih.gov/pubmed?term=Journal%20of%20Toxicology%20and%20Environmental%20Health%20sucralose, accessed April 30, 2012.

3   Joseph Mercola, DO, "Avoiding Artificial Sweeteners? This Study Will Surprise You." http://articles.mercola.com/sites/articles/archive/2011/09/20/why-are-millions-of-americans-getting-this-synthetic-sweetener-in-their-drinking-water.aspx?e_cid=20110920_DNL_art_1, accessed September 20, 2011.

4   Lynne Melcombe, *Health Hazards of White Sugar* (Vancouver, BC: Alive Books, 2002).

5   Randall Fitzgerald, *The Hundred-Year Lie* (New York: Plume, 2007).

6   Karen Evans and Doris Sarjeant, *Hard to Swallow* (New York: Alive Books, 1998).

7   K. S. Collison, "Dietary trans fats combined with monosodium glutamate induces dyslipidemia and impairs spatial memory," *Physiology & Behavior,* March 3, 2010. http://www.ncbi.nlm.nih.gov/pubmed/19945473, accessed April 30, 2012.

8   Lita Lee, PhD, and Lisa Turner with Burton Goldberg, *The Enzyme Cure* (Tiburon, CA: Future Medicine Publishing, Inc., 1998), p. 233.

9   Russell Blaylock, MD, *Excitotoxins: The Taste That Kills* (Albuquerque, NM: Health Press, 1996).

10   Lee and Turner with Goldberg, *The Enzyme Cure,* p. 235.

11   Jillian Boyle, "Start 2004 Slim!" *Woman's World,* December 30, 2003.

Chapter 4

1   Johnny Bowden, PhD, CNS, *The 150 Healthiest Foods on Earth* (Beverly, MA: Fair Winds Press, 2007), p. 55.

2   Ann Louise Gittleman, MS, CNS, *The Fat Flush Plan* (New York: McGraw-Hill, 2002), p. 35.

3   Michelle Schoffro Cook, PhD, *Healing Injuries the Natural Way* (Toronto, ON: Your Health Press, 2004), p. 47.

4   Sandra Cabot, MD, "Fatty Liver." http://www.liverdoctor.com/index.php?page=liver-problems&subpage=fatty-liver&gclid=CLGk1qC4m6sCFSUaQgod9ECVjA, accessed September 13, 2011.

5   Frances Sheridan Goulart, *Super Healing Foods* (Paramus, NJ: Reward Books, 1985), p. 88.

6   M. A. Wien et al. "Almonds vs. complex carbohydrates in weight reduction program," *International Journal of Obesity and Related Metabolic Disorders: Journal of the International Association for the Study of Obesity,* November 2003. http://www.ncbi.nlm.nih.gov/pubmed/14574348, accessed April 30, 2012.

7   Brenda Kearns, "Gained Weight This Winter?" *Woman's World,* March 2, 2004.

8   Brenda Kearns, "Superfood Discovery," *First for Women,* June 9, 2008, pp. 30–33.

9   Morten, Georg Jensen, "Acute effect of alginate-based preload on satiety feelings, energy intake, and gastric emptying rate in healthy subjects," *Obesity,* July 21, 2011. http://www.ncbi.nlm.nih.gov/pubmed/21779093, accessed April 30, 2012.

10   Bruce Fife, ND, *The Coconut Miracle* (Wayne, NJ: Avery Trade, 2004).

11   Edward Howell, *Enzyme Nutrition* (Wayne, NJ: Avery, 1985).

12   Kathleen Willcox and Helen Matatov, "The Enzyme Cure," *First for Women,* July 30, 2007, pp. 30–33.

13   Hiromi Shinya, *The Enzyme Factor* (San Francisco: Council Oak Books, 2005), p. 34.

14   Amy Capetta, "No Prescription Needed!" *Woman's World,* July 5, 2005.

15   "Fat-Burning Foods," *Woman's World,* April 27, 2004.

16   Gittleman, *The Fat Flush Plan,* p. 19.

17   Ibid., p. 35.

18   "Fat-Burning Foods," *Woman's World.*

19   Wien et al. "Almonds vs. complex carbohydrates in weight reduction program."

20   Gittleman, *The Fat Flush Plan,* p. 42.

21   "Fat-Burning Foods," *Woman's World.*

22   Ibid.

23   Ibid.

24   Ibid.

25   Kearns, "Superfood Discovery."

26   Steven Bolling et al., "Blueberry intake alters skeletal muscle and adipose tissue peroxisome proliferator-activated receptor activity and reduces insulin resistance in obese rats," *Journal of Medicinal Food,* December 2011. http://www.ncbi.nlm.nih.gov/pubmed/21861718, accessed April 30, 2012.

27   M. R. Ramirez et al., "Effect of lyophilised *vaccinium* berries on memory, anxiety, and locomotion in adult rats," *Pharmacological Research,* December 2005. http://www.ncbi.nlm.nih.gov/pubmed?term=anthocyanins%20short%20term%20memory, accessed September 6, 2012.

28   Michelle Schoffro Cook, PhD, *The Phytozyme Cure* (Toronto, ON: John Wiley & Sons, 2010).

29   Kearns, "Superfood Discovery."

30   Caitlin Castro, "Eat One of These a Day—And Lose 20 Lbs Fast," *Woman's World,* August 26, 2003.

31   Leslie Beck, "Food for Thought: Is Your Stomach or Your Head Guiding You to Overeat?" *Globe and Mail,* 2011.

32   Castro, "Eat One of These a Day."

33   H. Ahmad et al., "Citrus limonoids and flavonoids: Enhancement of phase II detoxification enzymes and their potential in chemoprevention," *Potential Health Citrus,* American Chemistry Society Symposium Series 936 (2006): 130–143.

34   Ibid.

35   A. Lyra et al., "Intestinal Microbiota and Overweight," *Beneficial Microbes.* http://www.ncbi.nlm.nih.gov/pubmed/21831779, accessed April 30, 2012.

36   E. Scarpellini et al., "Gut microbiota and obesity," *Internal and Emergency Medicine,* October 2010. http://www.ncbi.nlm.nih.gov/pubmed/20865475, accessed April 30, 2012.

37   "Quinoa Health Benefits." http://www.naturopathycure.com/Quinoa-Health-Benefits. php, accessed September 6, 2012.

Chapter 5

1   Jillian Boyle, "Is Lymphatic Stress the Reason You're Fat? Bloated? Hungry for Junk Food?" *Woman's World*, March 2, 2004.

2   "Ask America's Ultimate Experts: I Can't Seem to Lose That Last 10 Pounds," *Woman's World*, May 19, 2008.

3   "Walk Off 20 Pounds by March!" *Woman's World*, January 26, 2009.

4   Jillian Boyle, "Start 2004 Slim!" *Woman's World*, December 30, 2003.

5   "Ask America's Ultimate Experts."

6   Brenda Kearns, "Gained Weight This Winter? Here's How to Get Rid of It," *Woman's World*, March 2, 2004.

7   William C. Dement, MD, PhD, *The Promise of Sleep* (New York: Bantam Dell, 2000).

8   Alan R. Hirsch, MD, FACP, *Scentsational Weight Loss* (New York: Touchstone, 1998).

9   Ann Louise Gittleman, MS, CNS, *The Fat Flush Plan* (New York: McGraw-Hill, 2002).

10 Jennifer Joseph, "Break the Yeast–Belly Fat Cycle," *Woman's World*, September 6, 2010.

11 Ibid.

12 Lita Lee, PhD, and Lisa Turner with Burton Goldberg, *The Enzyme Cure* (Tiburon, CA: Future Medicine Publishing, Inc., 1998), p. 237.

13 C. M. Denzer and J. C. Young, "The effect of resistance exercise on the thermic effect of food," *International Journal of Sport Nutrition and Exercise Metabolism*, September 2003. http://www.ncbi.nlm.nih.gov/pubmed/14669938, accessed September 6, 2012.

14 "Walk Off 20 Pounds by March!"

15 "A Brief Review of Some of the Research Evidence on the Effectiveness of Hypnosis." http://tomlinsonhypnosis.com/Jan2011/hypnostats.pdf, accessed September 6, 2012.

16 Vinoth K. Ranganathan et al., "From mental power to muscle power; gaining strength by using the mind," *Neuropsychologia* 42, 2004.

17 Candace Pert, PhD, *Molecules of Emotion: The Science Behind Mind-Body Medicine* (New York: Simon & Schuster, 1999).

18 Frances Albrecht, MS, CN, PhD, "The Basics of Detoxing Your Liver," *Healthwell*, April 1997.

19 Michelle Schoffro Cook, PhD, *The 4-Week Ultimate Body Detox Plan* (Toronto, ON: John Wiley & Sons, 2004), pp. 227–228.

20 Gabrielle Lichterman, "Make This Your Slimmest Summer!" *Woman's World*.

Chapter 6

1   *Woman's World*, December 18, 2008.

2   H. J. Park et al., "Combined effects of genistein, quercetin, and resveratrol in human and 3T3-L1 adipocytes," *Journal of Medicinal Food*, December 2008.

3   Akira Niijima and Katsuya Nagai, "Effect of olfactory stimulation with flavor of grapefruit oil and lemon oil on the activity of sympathetic branch in the white adipose tissue of the epididymis," *Experiential Biological Medicine*, 2003.

4   A. Bhattacharya, "Conjugated linoleic acid and chromium lower body weight and visceral fat mass in high-fat-diet-fed mice," *Lipids*, May 2006. http://www.ncbi.nlm.nih.gov/pubmed/16933788, accessed May 1, 2012.

5   Ibid.

6   "The Slimming Pill That Prevents Heart Attacks, Diabetes, and the Blues!" *Woman's World*, July 13, 2009.

7   Amy Capetta, "No Prescription Needed!" *Woman's World*, July 5, 2005.

8   Ibid.

9   Barbara Smalley, "The Belly Fat Solution," *Woman's World*, July 29, 2003.

10   Alan R. Hirsch, MD, FACP, *Scentsational Weight Loss* (New York: Touchstone, 1998).

11   "Science of Scent." http://www.health-vitality.com/weightloss/article.htm, accessed July 21, 2011.

12   Ibid.

13   S. Warrenburg, "Effects of fragrance on emotions: mood and physiology," *Chemical Senses*, January 2005 Supplement. www.ncbi.nlm.nih.gov/pubmed/15738139, accessed November 27, 2012.

14   A. R. Hirsch, MD, FACP, "Smell and Sexual Arousal," *Encyclopedia of Food Science and Technology, Second Edition* (New York: John Wiley & Sons, Inc., 1999), pp. 81–7.

15   E. Scarpellini et al., "Gut microbiota and obesity," *Internal and Emergency Medicine*, October 2010. http://www.ncbi.nlm.nih.gov/pubmed/20865475, accessed May 1, 2012.

16   M. Tamura et al., "Effects of probiotics on allergic rhinitis induced by Japanese cedar pollen: Randomized double-blind, placebo-controlled clinical trial, *International Archives of Allergy and Immunology*, December 2007. http://www.ncbi.nlm.nih.gov/pubmed/17199093, accessed September 6, 2012.

17   P. D. Cani et al., "Involvement of gut microbiota in the development of low-grade inflammation and type 2 diabetes associated with obesity," *Gut Microbes*, July 2012. http://www.ncbi.nlm.nih.gov/pubmed/22572877, accessed September 6, 2012.

18   M. W. Hull and P. L. Beck, "Clostridium difficile-associated colitis," *Canadian Family Physician*, November 2004. http://www.ncbi.nlm.nih.gov/pubmed?term=probiotics%20colitis%20british%20columbia, accessed September 10, 2012.

19   R. D'Arienzo et al., "Immunomodulatory effects of *Lactobacillus casei* administration in a mouse model of gliaden-sensitive enteropathy," *Scandinavian Journal of Immunology*, October 2011. http://www.ncbi.nlm.nih.gov/pubmed/21615450, accessed September 10, 2012.

20   L. Pineda Mde et al., "A randomized, double-blind, placebo-controlled pilot study of probiotics in active rheumatoid arthritis," *Medical Science Monitor*, June 2011. http://www.ncbi.nlm.nih.gov/pubmed?term=rheumatoid%20arthritis%20university%20of%20western%20probiotic, accessed September 10, 2012.

21   U. Hoppu et al., "Probiotics and dietary counselling targeting maternal dietary fat intake modifies breast milk fatty acids and cytokines," *European Journal of Nutrition*, March 2012. http://www.ncbi.nlm.nih.gov/pubmed/21626296, accessed September 10, 2012.

22   P. Mastromarino et al., "Antiviral activity of *Lactobacillus brevis* towards herpes simplex virus type 2: Role of cell wall associated components," *Anaerobe*, December 2011. http://www.ncbi.nlm.nih.gov/pubmed/21621625, accessed September 10, 2012.

23 M. Popova et al., "Beneficial effects of probiotics in upper respiratory tract infections and their mechanical actions to antagonize pathogens," *Journal of Applied Microbiology*, July 2012. http://www.ncbi.nlm.nih.gov/pubmed/22788970, accessed September 10, 2012.

24 J. Feher et al., "Role of gastrointestinal inflammations in the development and treatment of depression," *Orvosi Hetilap*, September 2011. http://www.ncbi.nlm.nih.gov/pubmed/21893478, accessed September 10, 2012.

25 Michelle Schoffro Cook, PhD, *The Brain Wash* (Toronto: John Wiley & Sons Canada, 2007), p. 93.

26 E. P. Iakovenko et al., "Effects of probiotic bifiform on efficacy of *Helicobacter pylori* infection treatment," *Therapeutic Archives*, 2006. http://www.ncbi.nlm.nih.gov/pubmed/16613091, accessed September 10, 2012.

27 E. Guilllemard et al., "Consumption of a fermented dairy product containing the probiotic *Lactobacillus casei* DN114001 reduces the duration of respiratory infections in the elderly in a randomised controlled trial," *British Journal of Nutrition*, January 2010. http://www.ncbi.nlm.nih.gov/pubmed/19747410, accessed September 10, 2012.

28 J. L. Rosenblum et al., "Calcium and vitamin D supplementation is associated with decreased abdominal visceral adipose tissue in overweight and obese adults," *American Journal of Clinical Nutrition*, January 2012.

29 I. J. Onakpoya et al., "Efficacy of calcium supplementation for management of overweight and obesity: Systematic review of randomized clinical trials," *Nutrition Review*, June 2011.

30 K. Décordé et al., "Chardonnay grape seed procyanidin extract supplementation prevents high-fat diet-induced obesity in hamsters by improving adipokine imbalance and oxidative stress markers," *Molecular Nutrition and Food Research*, May 2009. http://www.ncbi.nlm.nih.gov/pubmed/19035554.

31 Robert Crayhon, MS, "The Ultimate Weight Loss Nutrient," *Total Health Resource Guide: Healthy Weight Management*, July/August 2002, pp. 11–12.

32 Ibid.

33 Ibid, p. 12.

34 Brenda Kearns, "Superfood Discovery," *First*, June 9, 2008, pp. 30–33.

35 L. A. Voloboueva et al., "(R)-alpha-lipoic acid protects retinal pigment epithelial cells from oxidative damage," *Investigative Ophthalmology and Visual Science*, November 2005. http://www.ncbi.nlm.nih.gov/pubmed/16249512, accessed May 1, 2012.

36 J. Liu et al., "Memory loss in old rats is associated with brain mitochondrial decay and RNA/DNA oxidation: Partial reversal by feeding acetyl-L-carnitine and/or R-alpha lipoic acid," *Proceedings of the National Academy of Sciences of the United States of America*, February 19, 2002. http://www.ncbi.nlm.nih.gov/pubmed/11854529, accessed May 1, 2012.

37 Andrea Marshall, "Milk Thistle Benefits Are Due to Silymarin." http://ezinearticles.com/?Milk-Thistle-Benefits-Are-Due-to-Silymarin&id=2186050, accessed March 29, 2010.

Index

Underscored references indicate boxed text.